T0021159

LOWER BLOOD PRESSURE WITHOUT DRUGS

Other Health Books by Roger Mason

The Natural Prostate Cure

The Minerals You Need

What is Beta Glucan?

Lower Cholesterol without Drugs

The Natural Diabetes Cure

Natural Health for Women

Macrobiotics for Everyone

Testosterone Is Your Friend

The Supplements You Need

LOWER BLOOD PRESSURE WITHOUT DRUGS

Curing Your Hypertension Naturally

THIRD EDITION

ROGER MASON

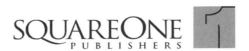

SQUAREONE PUBLISHERS

The information and advice contained in this book are based upon the research and the personal and professional experiences of the author. They are not intended as a substitute for consulting a healthcare professional. The publisher and author are not responsible for any adverse effects or consequences resulting from the use of any of the suggestions, preparations, or procedures discussed in this book. All matters pertaining to your physical health should be supervised by a healthcare professional. It is a sign of wisdom, not cowardice, to seek a second or third opinion.

Cover Designer: Jeannie Rosado
In-House Editor: Erica Shur
Typesetter: Gary A. Rosenberg

Square One Publishers
115 Herricks Road
Garden City Park, NY 11040
(516) 535-2010 • (877) 900-BOOK

Library of Congress Cataloging-in-Publication Data
Names: Mason, Roger, 1946– author.
Title: Lower blood pressure without drugs / Roger Mason.
Description: Third edition. | Garden City Park, NY : Square One Publishers [2019] | Includes index.
Identifiers: LCCN 2018049832 | ISBN 9780757004827
Subjects: LCSH: Hypertension—Alternative treatment. | Hypertension—Popular works. | Dietary supplements. | Naturopathy.
Classification: LCC RC685.H8 M294 2019 | DDC 616.1/32—dc23
LC record available at https://lccn.loc.gov/2018049832

Copyright © 2020 by Roger Mason

All rights reserved. No part of this publication may be reproduced, scanned, uploaded, stored in a retrieval system, or transmitted, in any form or by any means, electronic, mechanical, photocopying, photoediting, recording, or otherwise, without the prior written permission of the publisher.

Printed in the United States of America

10   9   8   7   6   5   4   3   2   1

Contents

About This Book

This book is the most researched, comprehensive, factual, and effective book in print on lowering blood pressure in print. Here you will find endless scientific, international, published clinical proof of everything you read. The vast majority of books on hypertension are simply full of misinformation. You don't lower blood pressure by covering up the symptoms taking toxic, expensive drugs with serious side effects. These poisons shorten your life, and hurt the quality of your life.

Using natural medicine, you treat the very cause of your problems with diet and lifestyle. *Diet and lifestyle cure disease.* Diet and lifestyle lower your blood pressure. Diet and lifestyle are the only real cure. Diet, proven supplements, natural hormones, exercise, weekly fasting, refusing prescription drugs and medical treatments, and ending any bad habits (like coffee) is the only path to wellness.

Americans have the highest blood pressure levels of anyone on earth. This is not merely due to stress. The key to understanding high blood pressure more than anything else is *insulin resistance.* Here our insulin loses effectiveness. *The main cause of this is our extreme consumption of various sugars and sugar substitutes.* Americans, on the average, hog down over 160 pounds of various sugars and sugar substitutes every year. Other major factors include obesity, lack of exercise, excessive fat and protein intake, and alcohol use. We are overfed and undernourished.

Essential hypertension is the most prevalent medical condition on the face of the earth. Over 65 million—one-third—of American adults have high blood pressure, defined as 140/90. Over 40 million more are pre-hypertensive, defined as pressures over 120/80. This is simply inexcusable. Anti-hypertensive drugs are the third most common prescription written. These toxic dangerous drugs simply make you worse. Yes, one third of all American adults suffer from high blood pressure, and many of them go undiagnosed. *Coronary heart disease (CHD) is the biggest killer of all worldwide.* This epidemic is completely unnecessary.

This book is based on the last thirty years of international published clinical research. Everything you need to know is in this factual, easy to read book. Be your own doctor, and take responsibility for your health.

1. About Hypertension

igh blood pressure is the most epidemic disease on earth bar none. No other medical condition approaches essential hypertension in numbers. In America alone there are over 100 million adults with pre-hypertension, or outright hypertension. This is classically defined as 140/90 readings. Pre-hypertension is defined as 130/85. You have to go beyond these readings and know other parameters. Total cholesterol, triglycerides, uric acid, CRP, homocysteine, insulin, blood sugar, GTT, albumin, creatinine, SGOT/AST, SGPT/ALT, and bilirubin are the twelve most important ones.

Surprisingly, you will find high blood pressure levels even in third world countries. This includes rural areas, where you would least expect it. A good example is the rural Nigerian people, who have little obesity, diabetes, or cholesterol problems, and smoking and coffee are not regular habits. Thirty percent of Nigerian adults are hypertensive, even though, ironically, they have a very low incidence of CHD (coronary heart disease). This is more proof that we cannot reduce the problem down to stress, since there is usually little stress in such rural people.

Age

Age is the most important factor of all, because everyone gets old—if they're lucky. There is a direct correlation between age and incidence of hypertension. The older you get, the higher your pressures generally. In developed countries, however, we are finding more and more problems with younger and younger people. We are finding increasing problems with obesity, diabetes, high cholesterol, and other such problems previously only associated with aging. We are now finding hypertension even in children and adolescents.

Insulin Resistance

You'll find by reading this book the main cause of hypertension is *insulin resistance.* Here, the body cells no longer respond well to normal amounts of insulin. This is basically caused by our outrageous intake of over 160 pounds of various sugars and sugar substitutes every year—more sugars per capita than any other country eats.

Kidney Conditions and Dysfunctions

Second to blood sugar dysmetabolism are various kidney conditions and dysfunctions. These are basically caused by our intake of twice the protein we need, nearly all of which is animal, not plant, protein. Excessive added table salt adds to this problem, but is highly overrated as a cause. Minerals are vital here, too, as we are very mineral deficient. We are overfed and undernourished. Kidney problems start as micro-albuminuria, then progress to clinical proteinuria, to progressive chronic renal failure, to outright kidney disease.

The Liver

The liver is also involved in blood pressure regulation. The liver is our largest internal organ (technically our skin is our largest organ), and controls blood sugar by the release of glycogen into the blood. Liver problems are also strongly associated with blood pressure. SGPT/ALT, SGOT/AST, and bilirubin levels are routinely checked during any comprehensive blood analysis. Liver problems are far too common in America due to three factors, 1) our 42 percent intake of saturated fats, 2) our over-consumption of alcohol, and 3) our inordinate intake of prescription and recreational drugs. Hypertension is clearly associated with elevated liver enzymes and fatty liver. Low bilirubin levels are common in hypertensive people.

Obesity

Obesity is a pillar of hypertension, and most patients are overweight. *One-in-three American adults are now clinically obese*, and obesity is a very powerful direct factor. *You must lose weight to lower blood pressure.*

Americans eat twice the food they need. We literally eat for two people every day. Men only need about 1,800 daily calories, and women only about 1,200. That's all. Calorie restriction greatly improves blood pressures, not only through weight loss, but by less oxidative stress from overeating. The University of Colorado found low calorie diets (from low fat foods) lowered blood pressure in people with no other lifestyle changes.

Oxidative Stress

Oxidative stress is also a major factor, where excessive free radicals cause damage to the entire body. We get almost no exercise anymore, and you must exercise to cure any kind of coronary or blood sugar condition. The answer to oxidative stress is better diet, fewer calories, regular exercise, and proven supplements—especially antioxidants. Oxidative stress can be measured by MDA (malondialdehyde) or TBARS (thiobarbituric acid) blood levels, but this is not necessary at all. Seoul University in Korea found poor antioxidant status (TAS) and oxidative stress to be basic causes of high blood pressure, and correlated strongly with obesity. Doctors at the University of Montreal discovered the development of insulin resistance and the model of hypertension, found to be prevented by chronic antioxidant therapies. *Oxidative stress is a major pathogenic factor in hypertension.*

America and Japan are the most stressful countries in the world, but this simply does not explain our current epidemic. Happy people have lower blood pressure. Healthy people have lower blood pressure. Happy marriages make for lower blood pressure. Loneliness is strongly associated with hypertension, and many people are lonely, especially the elderly, widowed, and divorced. Happiness and satisfaction with your job or vocation are also factors. Owning a pet, especially a dog, means lower blood pressure. People who go to church regularly and are spiritually minded, have lower blood pressure. Psychological and emotional issues of all kinds also raise blood pressure. It's not just stress.

Treatments

Most all doctors recommend one of five classes of dangerous, toxic drugs that cover up a symptom, and make your health worse. This ever changing array of pharmaceutical poisons includes diuretics, beta blockers, ACE inhibitors, angiotensin II receptor antagonists, and calcium channel blockers. Tens of billions of dollars of these toxins are sold worldwide every year, especially in America. This parade of dangerous chemicals changes constantly; popular ones disappear, while new ones are promoted as the "Magic Answer" to hypertension. One is far better off *doing absolutely nothing,* rather than taking these. They falsely trick the body into lowering pressures, and do not add to quality or length of life. Quite the opposite!

We will not discuss hypotension, or low blood pressure per se, for various reasons. This is very rare compared to high blood pressure. There is almost no research in the international clinical literature on this condition. The bottom line here is that *you can cure low blood pressure the very same way as high blood pressure.* Diet, exercise, supplements, hormones, fasting (if possible), no prescription drugs, and ending any bad habits should cure this in six months or less. If someone has a weak heart, or is very elderly, the results will be less dramatic of course.

Conditions Associated With Hypertension

Hypertension does not merely mean poor quality of life and early death. Many, many medical conditions are associated with it. Heart disease is the biggest killer of all by far. *Hypertension exacerbates any heart or artery problem.* Hypertension predisposes one to an endless litany of diseases, such as various cancers and diabetes. Studies have shown it is the major cause of erectile dysfunction (ED) in men. There is a very high incidence of ED in hypertensives. High blood pressure contributes to Alzheimer's, senility, mental decline, loss of memory, sleep disorders, lack of energy, poor cognition and other problems as we age. Sleep disorders are clearly correlated with hypertension, metabolic syndrome, and insulin resistance. The National Institute on Ageing links dementia as directly correlated with higher blood pressure. The Third National Health and Nutrition Survey found that the higher the blood pressure the poorer the cognitive performance in people over 60.

Biological And Psychological Racial Differences

Political correctness tells us there are no differences between the races other than skin color. Scientists, however, know there are countless biological and psychological racial differences. People of African heritage in America, but not in Africa, have epidemic rates of hypertension, diabetes, heart disease, prostate cancer, breast cancer, and other conditions. Latinos in America are more susceptible to insulin resistance and subsequent hypertension, but not in their native countries. All these factors lead to shorter life spans for people of color. To deny racial differences and not publish studies using race as a factor, hurts these people. It means they will not get the care and treatment they need, nor the preventive measures to avoid these unnecessary health conditions.

CONCLUSION

High blood pressure is the most prevalent medical condition on earth, common and dangerous, while the causes and cures are all too obvious. This is an unnecessary epidemic. The medical establishment promotes harmful, toxic, expensive options. The best cure for hypertension is a change in diet and lifestyle.

2. Diagnostics

How do we diagnose hypertension? How do you know if in fact you really have hypertension or pre-hypertension? What markers are most important? Certainly the most important and basic test is simply one's diastolic and systolic blood pressures. *If you are over 90 diastolic or 140 systolic, you are at risk. These are the accepted cutoff points,* 140 over 90 is the Magic Number. Of course, you would really rather be looking at levels of more like 120 over 80.

Pre-hypertension occurs when you get to a level near 130 over 85. If you are pre-hypertensive, always remember that an ounce of prevention is worth ten pounds of cure. Be proactive, and do something about it.

TESTING YOUR BLOOD PRESSURE

Beside one's diastolic and systolic blood pressures, there are other important markers to be taken into consideration.

Blood Sugar Level

Your blood sugar level is vital; know your fasting blood sugar level. *This should be 85 or less.* Do not accept the usual limit of "100 or less" from the medical conglomerate, no matter what your doctor tells you. It is an established fact *that sickness and mortality increase with any blood sugar level over 85.*

You can get an inexpensive and accurate **no-code home blood sugar meter** at the drugstore for $20. One problem is that some people have a normal blood sugar level, but they are still insulin-resistant.

If your level is over 85, definitely get a safe, accurate, inexpensive *Glucose Tolerance Test* (GTT). To test your blood sugar, drink a measured 75g cup of glucose solution, wait two hours, and test your blood sugar again. It should be 10 points under the accepted Western level, not the level the doctor will tell you. *Anything over this indicates insulin resistance.* The GTT is the gold standard here, but it is very underutilized. Even if your fasting glucose is 85 or less, you really should still get this inexpensive test done.

The *HbA1c* test is also excellent, and can show your blood sugar average over the past three months. *You should have a level of 4.6 percent or less.* This equates to a blood glucose level of 85. Do not accept the usual accepted values, 4.6 percent or less. You really don't need this test unless you are diabetic, pre-diabetic, or suspect you are diabetic. You can find inexpensive HbA1c tests in drugstores, on online labs without a doctor. This six month blood glycation (bonding to glucose) average is very reliable.

Fasting Plasma Or Serum Insulin

Along with blood sugar you should test your fasting plasma or serum insulin. This is a very inexpensive blood test. This can be done with online labs like www.healthlabs.com for 30 dollars without a doctor.

You want a serum fasting level of 5.0 µU/ml or less. Yes, you can do this. Knowing your insulin level is very important. Diet and lifestyle can lower this greatly.

Total Cholesterol And Triglycerides

Test your total cholesterol (TC) and triglycerides (TG). HDL (high-density lipoprotein) and LDL (low-density lipoprotein) levels are also useful, but it's not as necessary. Your TC and TG are far more important. *Your total cholesterol is the best indicator of all for heart and artery disease in general.*

Total Cholesterol

Some studies show good correlation of high TC and hypertension, and some don't. You must test your total cholesterol every year.

Inexpensive home tests are available on the Internet as well. Your total cholesterol should be about *150 or less*, not 200 or less as you're commonly told. *Mortality and sickness increase with any level over 150,* and especially over 200. American adults test at about 240 on the average. This is a major reason why heart disease of all kinds is so prevalent. Yes, this applies to all types of coronary heart disease. *You must keep your level around 150 for optimum health.*

Yes, this is a practical ideal, and billions of rural Asians and Africans prove it. They have only a fraction of the CHD conditions we do. However, if they move here and adopt the Western diet, they get just as much or more heart and artery disease.

High total cholesterol is basically due to intake of saturated animal fats from red meat, poultry, eggs, and dairy foods. Ten percent fish and seafood will not raise your levels. Cholesterol is only found in animal products. The best way to keep your cholesterol down is to stop eating these foods. Most people are unwilling to do this. You can eat 10 percent seafood if you like.

High Triglycerides

High triglycerides are far more important. Science agrees that triglycerides are a basic indicator of hypertension and CHD in general. *Your triglycerides should be 100 mg/dL or less.* Mortality and sickness increase with any level over 100, especially diabetes and other blood sugar disorders. High triglycerides are one of the very basic signs of hypertension.

High levels are generally due to excessive intake of any simple sugars, including fruit juice, honey, dried fruit, white sugar, and others. This includes sugar substitutes, such as sucralose, aspartame, and stevia. All natural sugars have the same effect, and honey is simply no better than white sugar. High TG is not due to fat intake like cholesterol is. Nearly all vegans and vegetarians have excessive intake of simple sugars, with resulting high TG levels. Your TG level must be less than 100. Limit your simple sugars and sugar substitute intake and you'll do fine.

C-reactive Protein

If you are over 40, it's a good idea to get your C-reactive protein (CRP) tested. This is an excellent and accurate marker of coronary heart disease (CHD) and chronic inflammation. High CRP is very clearly correlated to high blood pressure, and should be 0.1 to 0.3 mg/dl.

The researchers of the world are in agreement that CRP is a reliable marker of blood pressure. Sungkyunkwan University in South Korea found there was a significant positive association between blood pressure and CRP.

At the famous Brigham Hospital in Boston they found that CRP levels are associated with the future development of hypertension. This suggests that hypertension is part of an inflammatory disorder. Even children now suffer from high blood pressure.

At the University of Wittten in Germany, doctors said obese children demonstrated significantly higher levels of CRP compared to non-obese children.

The Shenzhen Hospital in China stated that plasma CRP level was positively correlated with glucose tolerance degree in essential hypertension patients.

Homocysteine

Homocysteine (Hcys) is also a very accurate marker of CHD events, but it is not as strong an indicator of high blood pressure. The evidence here is sometimes conflicting, but the positive studies far outweigh the negative. The bottom line is that *Hcys is a very basic and vital marker for heart and artery health in general.* You should still keep your Hcys level under 10 mmol, and preferably well under 10. You should definitely test this to know the status of your heart and artery health.

At Shanxi Hospital in China (*Zhonghua Laonian* v 8, 2006) they clearly saw, "A positive relationship was found between pulse pressure and homocysteine. This relationship remained after adjustment for classical essential hypertension risk factors."

At the Preventive Medical Center in Japan (*Hypertension Research* v 29, 2006) they said, "These data suggest that high plasma homocysteine is associated with increased systemic arterial stiffness, which may enhance blood pressure."

At Affiliated Hospital in China (*Shandong Yiyao* v 46, 2006) they found, "In conclusion, the attack of hypertension complicated by ischemic stroke in old patients had a relationship with the increase in plasma homocysteine." They suggested vitamin supplementation instead of drug therapy.

At General Hospital in Taiwan they concluded that hypertensive subjects had higher fasting plasma Hycs concentration and insulin resistance.

Some studies have found no relationship. This is irrelevant in that Hycs is a proven diagnostic marker for CHD, in general. Even if Hycs is not a completely reliable tool for hypertension, it is a time proven one for overall heart and artery diseases. This is a very important diagnostic tool. The famous Framingham Study found (*Hypertension* v 42, 2003) no major relationship with blood pressure. Another review of the Framingham Study (*Clinical Chemistry* v 41, 2003) said it was, "unproven."

Uric Acid

Uric acid is also very important. Only 15 percent of our blood uric acid is caused by the purines in our food, while 85 percent is endogenous and made by our bodies. Your level should be under 5 mg/dl. *Animal foods promote uric acid* due to animal proteins and saturated fat. Alcohol definitely promotes uric acid production. Our excessive intake of beef, pork, lamb, chicken, turkey, eggs, dairy products of all kinds, and organ meats causes high blood uric acid levels. You can eat fish and seafood in moderation (10 percent of your diet) if you so choose. High uric acid comes from eating animal foods, not purines.

Vegetarians and vegans simply don't have this problem. Have you ever heard of a vegetarian with gout or high uric acid levels? Lacto-ovo "vegetarians" who eat diary and/or eggs, yet call themselves "vegetarians," do have higher uric acid levels, even though there are no purines in dairy products or eggs. High uric acid is associated not only with gout (the most painful form of arthritis) but many other illnesses. You definitely want low uric acid levels. There is no uric acid in plant foods; *the problem is caused by the proteins and fats in animal foods.* This is why you limit fish and seafood to 10 percent of your diet if you don't want to be a vegetarian.

People in the highest quarter (quartile) of blood uric acid have three times the CHD death rate, compared to those in the lowest quarter. People in the highest quartile have over twice the all-cause mortality of those in the lowest quartile. Low uric acid is your ideal, and you can only attain this by avoiding or limiting meat, poultry, eggs, and dairy. *All dairy foods must go.*

At Osaka University (*European Journal of Epidemiology* v 18, 2003) the doctors concluded, "These results indicate that high serum uric acid level is closely associated with an increased risk for hypertension, and impaired fasting glucose or Type II diabetes."

At the Institute for Cardiology in Poland the doctors there found hypertensive patients showed increased serum uric acid levels and a higher incidence of hyperuricemia. The same results were found in Tottori University in Japan, Shangxi Medical University in China, Hiroshima University in Japan, Baylor College in Texas, and many other hospitals and clinics around the world.

At the University of Verona in Italy (*Metabolism, Clinical and Experimental* v 45, 1996) they found an astounding 88 percent of hypertensive subjects had high blood uric acid! This is stunning. At the Moscow Meditsina Klinicheskaya, 79 percent of hypertensives had high uric acid.

At the National Cardiovascular Center in Japan (*American Journal of Hypertension* v 15, 2002) patients were put on a healthier diet. This caused them to lose weight and lower their uric acid levels. This, of course, resulted in impressive reductions of their systolic and diastolic pressures. The famous Bogalusa Heart Study showed high uric acid levels were clearly and strongly correlated with hypertension, even in children.

The most impressive of all is the Framingham Heart Study. This is the longest and largest CHD study in history. The researchers there concluded, "In summary, serum uric acid level was an independent predictor of hypertension incidence . . ."

Kidney Function

Since the kidneys are so central to blood pressure regulation, there are two very important tests that diagnose kidney function. *Creatinine* (not to be confused with the amino acid creatine) is a very good indicator of kidney health. Values vary from lab to lab. If the range is, say, .8 to 1.3 mg/dl for men over 60, and .6 to 1.2 for women over 60, then you want to be right in those narrow ranges. There are no kidney specific supplements, so the answer here is *a low-protein diet* with no meat, poultry, eggs, or dairy, and only 10 percent seafood if you wish. Salt should be moderated, and high salt foods like pickles, salted chips, olives, and such should be avoided. There is no reason to go on an ultra-low salt diet, as explained in Chapter 9: The Low-Sodium Myth. You still must avoid excessive use of table salt.

A good kidney test to use along with creatinine is albumin (protein) in the urine, known as ***microalbuminuria***. Albumin-urea is highly correlated with arterial pressures. This is called urinary albumin excretion or UAE. It is tested by collecting urine for a period of time, such as 8 hours. Any reading more than 15 mcg per minute is considered proof of excessive excretion. There is also a spot test where any reading over 30 mcg per liter is evidence of damage. This shows kidney damage and is known as "incipient nephropathy."

At the University of Insubria (*American Journal of Hypertension* v 14, 2001) they said, "In conclusion, in never-treated hypertensive patients, microalbuminurea is not only associated with greater myocardial mass (enlarged heart), but is also related with preclinical impairment of LV (left ventricle) diastolic function." At the University of Pisa they found that microalbuminurea, accompanied by evidence of subclinical inflammation, is a strong correlate of metabolic abnormalities in essential hypertension. This identifies a patient subset at very high cardiovascular risk. At Sungkyunk-wan University in South Korea, they stated albumin and CRP were significantly higher in the hypertensive patients. At Brazil's Federal University, they found UAE rates correlated positively with systolic doctor's office blood pressure measurements and ambulatory blood pressure.

Kidney problems are caused by excess animal protein in the diet. This can only come from meat, poultry, eggs, and dairy consumption. Excess salt intake also stresses the kidneys, forcing them to constantly excrete the excess sodium to maintain the vital sodium-to-potassium balance. Hypertension is usually related to weak and damaged kidneys. There are a few people who are salt sensitive. This is *not* sodium chloride that causes their problems, but rather the impaired kidney function that can no longer maintain the sodium homeostasis in their blood. Such people *do* need to limit salt intake, because their impaired kidneys can't handle the load. This does not mean an obsessive low-salt diet with special foods at all, but merely the moderation of added salt to their food. Excess sodium comes from the salt shaker and salt processed foods. The proper treatment is a low-calorie, low-protein diet, and fast weekly until their kidneys strengthen and repair themselves.

Liver Function

The liver must be mentioned as well. The SGOT/AST and SGPT/ALT, along with bilirubin, are the three major indicators. The liver is central to blood sugar production from glycogen. Our livers are harmed by intake of fats (especially saturated animal fats), alcohol, and most all drugs, especially pharmaceuticals. Recreational drugs, even marijuana, should be dropped. A routine blood analysis will have these three levels listed along with their ranges.

CONCLUSION

High blood pressure is diagnosed and then treated to reduce the danger of developing a stroke, heart disease or heart failure, dementia, vascular disease, renal disease, or premature death. An early and correct diagnosis plays an important role in reducing the risk of these related cardiovascular diseases.

Buy an inexpensive blood pressure monitor and test yourself regularly. This is important, since usually there are no obvious symptoms associated with hypertension. As outlined in this chapter, high blood pressure can be cured with diet and lifestyle.

3. Insulin Resistance Is the Key

hy do some people raise their blood pressure, and others don't, when subjected to the same life situations? The answer is insulin resistance, more than any other factor. *This includes all blood sugar dysmetabolism in general.* Whenever you study hypertension, you find insulin resistance more than any other factor. There is a wealth of information on the action of insulin, blood sugar, metabolic syndrome, and insulin resistance as the basis for hypertension. This chapter will purposely cite quote studies to make the point as strongly as possible. You'll see overemphasis and repetition because this is so basic. This entire syndrome is prediabetic, and is epidemic in America. Much of this goes undiagnosed, and therefore untreated.

CAUSES OF BLOOD SUGAR PROBLEMS

Why are blood sugar problems so epidemic? There are four main causes, but the main cause is our extreme consumption of sugars and sugar substitutes. Americans stuff down over 160 pounds of various sugars every year that they don't need at all. Now they also eat toxic sugar substitutes like sucralose. It doesn't matter whether it's white sugar, raw sugar, brown sugar, fruit juice, dried fruit, corn syrup, honey, maple syrup, fructose, cane syrup, agave, molasses, or any other simple sugar—they are all basically the same. They all have the same negative effect on our health. Sugar substitutes, even natural ones like stevia, are just as bad or worse. Sugar is sugar is sugar.

Another reason is our severe lack of nutrition, especially minerals. We are all mineral deficient. We are overfed and undernourished. We eat twice the calories we need, but don't get the nutrients we need. Read Chapter 7: The Minerals You Need.

Lack of exercise is the third major reason. Very few people do any physical work anymore. The more exercise the better, whether it is aerobic or resistance. Read Chapter 12: You Must Exercise.

Obesity is the fourth major cause. One third of Americans are obese, and many of the rest are overweight. Obesity is not only strongly and directly related to blood pressure but to all-cause mortality as well. Read Chapter 6: Obesity Is Basic.

Even in a rural agrarian area, such as Nepal, a quarter of the adults are hypertensive. Even more have abnormal glucose metabolism. This was discovered at the University of Nepal in Katmandu. How can rural agrarian people with little stress in their lives have such an epidemic? This is common worldwide.

SCIENTIFIC RESEARCH

The entire world's scientific community is in basic agreement that *blood sugar dysmetabolism is at the heart of blood pressure conditions.* Let's look at some of the countless studies.

The University of Verona, in Italy, found fasting insulin was strongly related to body mass index, waist-to-hip and waist-to-thigh circumference ratios, serum lipids, and blood pressure. The Royal Victoria Hospital in England found insulin clearance was reduced in the hypertensive group.

Nerima General Hospital in Japan found that the most important determinant of systolic and diastolic blood pressures was the plasma insulin concentration. Ichihara College in Japan established that abnormal glucose tolerance (assessed by a 75 g oral GTT) had direct pathophysiological relevance to endothelial dysfunction in moderate hypertensive patients. Sapporo University in Japan (*Hypertension Research* v 18, 1995) reported, "The results indicate that 1) insulin sensitivity declines with age, and 2) insulin sensitivity is already diminished in early hypertension. Insulin sensitivity is low in patients with essential hypertension (EH)." Hiroshima University, in Japan, found that hypertension was positively associated with a significant elevation in BMI, triglycerides, uric acid, fasting glucose, fasting insulin, and GTT results, as well as a decrease in HDL.

At Taipei Veterans Hospital, in Taiwan, it was found that fasting insulin concentrations were significantly associated with systolic and diastolic pressures, after accounting for sex, BMI, and waist-to-hip ratio.

At UCLA they concluded insulin resistance was related to hypertension and blood pressure in subjects without diabetes.

At Middlesex Hospital in England the doctors very wisely suggested that a GTT should be a routine test for anyone over 40, and anyone who suspects a blood sugar issue. *This is true even with a normal fasting blood sugar level.* Much of insulin resistance goes undiagnosed, and the GTT is severely underused.

At Joujinkai Hemodialysis Clinic, in Japan, they stated very clearly that hypertension is caused by metabolic syndrome. Remember that the accepted definition of insulin resistance is much less strict than in the real world, just like the blood sugar, cholesterol, and triglyceride levels. The real world incidence for this is much higher than reported. Again, at the same facility they found that insulin resistance seems to have a closer relationship to blood pressure than does plasma insulin per se.

At Japan Cardiovascular Center, it was concluded that insulin resistance, rather than hyperinsulemia, is closely associated to essential hypertension. At Sungkyunkwan University their results showed that insulin resistance, body mass index, and waist circumference are independent risk factors of a high blood pressure in South Koreans. Clearly obesity is 1) strongly correlated with insulin resistance, and 2) a strong factor in hypertension per se.

At the Italian Institute Auxologico, the doctors found that systolic blood pressure correlates significantly with both fasting plasma glucose (FPG) and glucose levels measured 2 hours after an oral glucose ingestion (2-h PG), even after adjustment for age and obesity. Furthermore, lean men with impaired fasting glucose (IFG) had a double multivariate-adjusted risk of hypertension compared to those with normal FPG.

At Huddinge Hospital, in Sweden, they suggested a routine GTT, since blood sugar levels are often normal in those with insulin resistance.

Three studies from Poland are clear. At the Academy of Medicine it was found that *the mean values of insulin levels were, in every case, elevated in patients with essential hypertension.* The Tetniczego Academy concluded that patients with hypertension had lower insulin sensitivity. The Endocrinology Clinic found the mean concentration of blood glucose was higher in patients with essential hypertension.

Much research has come from China. At First Hospital insulin resistance appeared in essential hypertension patients with impaired glucose tolerance and (or) hyperinsulemia. At the Shandong Hospital doctors said that the levels of fasting glucose, insulin, and total cholesterol in the hypertension group were significantly higher than those of the controls. At Xi'an Medical University it was noted that essential hypertension is correlated with a metabolic disturbance characterized by insulin resistance. At Quingdao Medical College, the results suggested that the synthesis and release of insulin were increased in the essential hypertension patients. General Naval Hospital found impaired glucose tolerance, hyperlipidemia, obesity, hyperinsulemia, and insulin resistance in patients with hypertension. At Yangzhou Medical College, the patients with hypertension and simple obesity had significantly higher levels of plasma glucose and insulin than normal. At Beijing's Friendship Hospital the doctors concluded that age, sex, BMI, fasting and 2 hour GTT glucose, and insulin levels were all positively related to blood pressure. At First Affiliated Hospital they also suggested using a routine GTT with all suspected hypertensives.

CURING INSULIN RESISTANCE

How do we cure insulin resistance? Eat a whole grain based diet, with no added sweets or sugars of any kind as much as possible. Limit fruit intake to 10 percent of your diet. Do not eat desserts, dried fruits, or drink fruit juice. Do not use sugar substitutes like stevia or sucralose. Studies have shown these are just as harmful (or worse) as regular simple sugars. In fact, you don't even need fruit in your diet. Read the article *Fruit Has Almost No Nutrition* on our website for more information. *Fruit is basically sugar (sucrose and fructose), water, and some fiber, with almost no vitamins, minerals, or other nutrients worth mentioning.*

Eat two meals a day. Fast one day a week. Limit intake of meat, poultry, and eggs if you insist on eating them. *Take dairy foods out of your life completely*, as all adults of all races are lactose intolerant. Casein (milk protein) is a proven cancer promoter.

Take proven supplements like lipoic acid, beta glucan, and CoQ10. Take a good mineral supplement with seventeen elements in the amounts you need. Insulin is a basic hormone, and all our hormones work harmoniously together in concert as a team. Balance all your other basic hormones, so your insulin will be as effective as possible.

Exercise regularly to burn off any excess sugar. *You must exercise to cure any blood sugar condition.* You will lose weight without trying, while eating all you want, if you just do these simple things. Follow a total program of diet and lifestyle, and nothing less. Diet is everything, also supplements, hormones, fasting, exercise, no prescription drugs, and no bad habits.

CONCLUSION

Insulin resistance, along with other blood sugar dysmetabolism, is the basic cause of high blood pressure. The cause of this is our extreme overconsumption of sugars and sugar substitutes, and poor diet in general. The next chapter discusses how whole grains are beneficial in controlling hypertension and blood sugar conditions.

4. Whole Grains— The Staff of Life

Whole grains are the very basis of your diet. Americans, however, eat a mere 1 percent of whole grains of their daily fare. This should be at least 50 percent. Brown rice, oatmeal, polenta, whole wheat and brown rice pasta, whole grain breads, barley, whole wheat couscous, corn meal, buckwheat, rye, and other whole grains should literally be your staff of life . The word "cereal" comes from the Roman goddess Ceres. Man became free from hit-or-miss survival when he developed agriculture, rather than just hunting and gathering. Grains have been the staple food of nearly all cultures throughout history. This is the difference between cavemen and those who created their own destiny. The rural Okinawans are the ultimate example here. They live the longest, and are the healthiest of all cultures. Whole grains are their staple.

TYPES OF WHOLE GRAINS

Let's look at the basic grains of the world.

- Rice is the most consumed food on the face of the earth. It is simply incomprehensible that most all people take the time, trouble, effort, and expense to refine rice, wheat, corn, and other grains to remove the valuable bran and other nutrients.

Brown rice should be the center of your meals. You can get brown rice pasta as well. Brown rice flour is very versatile. Sweet brown rice is available, but is meant more for desserts than an entree. Wild rice is really a grass, not a grain. Its distinct flavor makes it better to mix with brown rice.

- Wheat is the second most consumed food for over six billion people. Bulgur is steamed whole wheat that has been presoaked. You can find whole wheat couscous if you look. Whole wheat and whole grain breads are staple foods.

- Corn is the third most popular grain. Corn on the cob is a basic food, as are corn kernels. (Frozen corn kernels are perfectly acceptable.) Fine corn flour is known as masa. Most all grits are refined. Course whole corn meal makes polenta when you add 3 cups of liquid for every cup of meal. There are corn pastas, but they tend to fall apart.

- Oats are generally only eaten as hot oatmeal for breakfast. Oat flakes go well in multigrain breads.

- Barley is a fine grain, and can be eaten as an entrée like rice, and not just limited to barley soup and making beer.

- Buckwheat has a distinctive taste, and can be mixed with other grains.

- Rye has a very strong flavor and is best used in multigrain breads.

- Millet is a staple in some countries, but little is used here. It can be used just like rice.

- Spelt, teff, and quinoa (KEEN-wah) are ancient grains that cost a little more, are very good, but are not well known.

- Sorghum is a powerful healing grain that is popular in some countries, but it just doesn't taste as good as other grains. It can be popped like popcorn and is delicious. It can also be mixed with other tastier grains.

You are dealing with insulin resistance and glycemic control more than anything. A whole grain based diet is the means to control these.

SCIENTIFIC RESEARCH

At Yonsei University in South Korea (*Atherosclerosis, Thrombosis, and Vascular Biology* v 21, 2001) patients were fed a whole grain based diet for just 16 weeks. *Their blood glucose fell an amazing 24 percent and their insulin levels 14 percent!* Lipid peroxidation (oxidized blood fats) fell 28 percent, which means less heart disease. This was done without any other treatments, just better diet. *Diet is the cure for insulin resistance and hypertension.*

At the U.S. Department of Agriculture (*Journal of the American College of Nutrition* v 19, 2000) they reported, "Consumption of, and number of, grains has been reported to control or improve glucose tolerance and reduce insulin resistance. A number of whole grain foods are beneficial in reducing insulin resistance and improvement in glucose tolerance." They suggest eating more whole grains, since Americans eat them as only 1 percent in their diet.

Researchers at Shaheed University in Tehran (*European Journal of Clinical Nutrition* v 59, 2005) studied 827 men and women. They concluded, "Whole grain intake is inversely, and refined grain intake is positively, associated with the risk of having metabolic syndrome. Recommendations to increase whole grain intake may reduce this risk." This was a very professionally done study.

At world renowned Harvard University (*American Journal of Clinical Nutrition* v 75, 2002) insulin sensitivity was improved greatly with the addition of whole grains to the diet. "Insulin sensitivity may be an important mechanism whereby whole grains reduce the risk of type 2 diabetes and heart disease." They suggested, "People should be encouraged to replace the refined grain foods in their diet, such as white bread and bagels, refined grain breakfast cereals, and white rice with whole grain choices." The researchers found that insulin sensitivity improved in a group of obese adults when they ate a diet rich in whole grain foods, such as brown rice, oats, barley, and corn. The conclusion was, "Whole grain foods may have favorable effects on insulin sensitivity. These effects may reduce the risk of type 2 diabetes and heart disease." Whole grains significantly increased insulin sensitivity and lowered insulin levels. This resulted in lower blood pressure of course.

At Simmons College, in Boston, (*American Journal of Clinical Nutrition* v 76, 2002) they reviewed the Health Professionals Study of over 50,000 men and women for ten years. *The more whole grains the people ate, the healthier they were, the lower their blood pressure, and less diabetes.* In the same volume of *AJCN* from the U.S. Department of Agriculture (and Harvard and Tufts) almost 3,000 people were studied. Again, the more whole grains they ate the lower their blood pressure, the less heart disease and diabetes. "Increased intakes of whole grains may reduce disease risk by means of favorable effects on metabolic risk factors." Also in the *AJCN* (v. 86, 2007) Harvard did another study and reported, "The fiber and nutrients in whole grains help prevent high blood pressure." Each serving of daily whole grains lowered blood pressure a full 4 percent per decade.

Diabetes Care (v 27, 2004) published, "DASH Diet Improves Insulin Sensitivity as Well as Hypertension." The DASH (Dietary Approaches to Stop Hypertension) diet is much better than the standard American diet, and emphasizes whole grains, beans, vegetables, fruits, and low-fat dairy products. It is designed to be high in fiber and nutrients, but low in fat and any type of sugar. There have been many studies on the DASH diet. In this study, 52 people were put on this regimen and got up to 50 percent improvement in insulin sensitivity, while dramatically lowering blood pressure in six months. This is certainly going in the right direction, especially for the

American Diabetes Association. DASH would be a lot better without dairy products of course.

The University of Kuopio, in Finland, (*American Journal of Clinical Nutrition* v 77, 2003) found that the more whole grains people ate, the lower their blood pressure, and the less diabetes they suffered from. *"An inverse association between whole grain intake and type 2 diabetes was found."* The less whole grains people ate the more antihypertensive drugs they took. This was based on over 4,000 otherwise healthy people without diabetes.

Men and women (*Journal of the American Diabetic Association* v 106, 2006) were given whole grains for 17 weeks to see if this would improve their cardiovascular health. Both their systolic and diastolic pressures were strongly reduced, along with mean arterial pressure (MAP). Their total cholesterol, uric acid, blood glucose, and other parameters fell as well. *Whole grains are heart healthy.*

At Pennsylvania State University (*Science Daily* Feb. 11, 2008) the researchers said, "Consumption of whole grains has been associated with a lower body weight and lower blood pressure." For twelve weeks 50 obese men and women of all ages were asked to eat whole grain foods along with vegetables and fruits. They even ate a little low-fat dairy products, poultry, and meat. Their CRP fell an amazing 38 percent, and their blood pressure fell as well. *They lost 8 to 11 pounds while eating all they wanted.* Obesity is a big factor in hypertension as we have discussed. We need more such fine studies.

At the University of Minnesota (*Proceedings of the Nutrition Society* v 62, 2003) 160,000 men and women were studied. "There is accumulating evidence that whole grain consumption is associated with a reduced risk of type 2 diabetes, and may improve glucose control." People who ate the most whole grains had the least blood sugar conditions. This involves far too many people to argue with.

Make whole grains your main staple. This should be the very basis of your diet. Eat at least 50 percent whole grains every day.

Worldwide published scientific studies prove this conclusively.

CONCLUSION

As seen in the chapter, studies around the world show that people who eat the most whole grains live the longest, and have the best health and least disease. A diet rich in whole grains can help regulate your blood sugar and can lower the risk of cardiovascular disease. You don't need toxic, harmful, expensive prescription drugs. In the next chapter, diet is shown to be the cure for hypertension.

5. Diet, Diet, Diet

Diet is everything. Diet cures disease. Diet cures insulin resistance. Diet lowers blood pressure. All other factors are secondary to what you eat every day. You can lower your blood pressure with diet (and exercise) alone, without any supplements, fasting, or hormones. Without a whole grain based diet, nothing is going to help you very much. We eat twice the calories we need; two people could live comfortably on what one American eats every day. This is why we're the fattest nation on earth.

Americans eat an astounding 42 percent fat calories. This is nearly all saturated, artery-clogging saturated animal fat. We only need about 8 percent vegetable oils in our food, so this is more than 500 percent of what we need. *We eat twice the protein we need.* We also eat an incredible 160 pounds of various sugars and sugar substitutes every year that we have no need for whatsoever. This massive sugar intake is the main cause of insulin resistance. Refined grains are another cause. This excess protein we eat causes high uric acid levels and kidney disease, among other problems. Yet, despite gulping down twice the food they need every day, Americans are completely undernourished, and don't get the vital nutrients they need—*overfed and undernourished.* Twice the calories we need, but half the nutrition!

You should eat according to your environment and your genetics. If you are of tropical ancestry living in a tropical area, you can and should, eat tropical and subtropical foods like bananas, avocadoes, yams, breadfruit, papayas, mangoes, yucca, boniato, taro, and other tropical foods. If the same person of tropical ancestry moves to, say, Canada, they can no longer eat these. Their environment is now temperate despite their genetics— *genetics and environment.*

FOODS TO EAT OR NOT TO EAT

Nature provides us the right foods to be in harmony with our environment and genetics.

- *Whole grains are your main staple.* **Whole grains**, such as brown rice, whole wheat, corn, buckwheat, barley, and oats, should be the very basis of your diet. This is covered in the previous chapter.

- **Beans** are very similar to whole grains. Beans and legumes are inexpensive, low in fat, high in protein, high in nutrients, and very filling. A half cup of cooked beans only contains about 120 calories and 2 percent fat calories.

- By the way, **tofu** is a heavily refined food with little nutrition, and should only be used occasionally. There are a good variety of whole soy foods, such as sausage, burgers, beef flavor, chicken flavor, tempeh, and others.

- Most **vegetables** can be eaten except the Nightshades. They include potatoes, tomatoes, peppers, and eggplants. These contain the deadly alkaloid solanine (and tomatine in tomatoes). Avoid tropical vegetables, unless you are of tropical descent living in a tropical environment. Also limit foods high in oxalic acid, like spinach and chard. Americans eat far too few green and yellow vegetables. The Chinese are the masters of vegetable recipes.

- You should eat local **fruits**, but only about 10 percent of your diet. Fruits are mostly sugar and water, and have very little nutrition. That's right, there are almost no vitamins, minerals, or other nutrients in fruits. They are a very poor nutrition source. *You actually do not need to eat any fruit at all.* Take the concept of desserts out of your life. Most Asian cultures do not include desserts as part of their meals. You do not need desserts. Start your meal with a hot delicious hearty soup, instead of having dessert at the end.

- Ten percent of your diet can be **seafood** if you don't want to be a vegetarian or vegan, and you have no allergy to seafood. You can easily be a vegetarian or vegan on a macrobiotic diet. Our canine teeth are biological proof we can eat 10 percent seafood. Eat soups and salads made from macrobiotic ingredients for variety. Get some cookbooks—be creative.

- *All dairy foods have to go.* **Milk and dairy foods** are absolutely the worst possible choices. This includes the low-fat and no-fat varieties. Taking lactase tablets such as Lactaid® is also not the answer. Goat, buffalo, camel, zebra, yak, giraffe, or whale milk are all basically the same, as they all contain lactose and casein. There is a universal allergy in adults to lactose or milk sugar. No adult of any race can digest lactose after the age of three. We stop producing the enzyme lactase after that age. Lactose does not merely pass harmlessly through your digestive system, but causes serious problems. Asians, Africans, American Indians, and other races are hypersensitive to lactose. The milk protein casein is the second reason not to eat dairy products. Casein is proven to promote various cancers, diabetes, coronary heart disease, and other such illnesses. The best discussion of this is found in Colin Campbell's book, *The China Study*. Here, he proves beyond any doubt that *the intake of animal proteins per se causes high disease rates and early death.* This is in addition to the saturated fats and cholesterol. Hard and soft cheeses are almost devoid of lactose but full of casein and saturated fat. Yogurt is not a health food, and never has been, as it is full of lactose and casein.

- **Fats and oils** should only be 10 to 20 percent of your diet, and from vegetable sources. *The Magic Number here is 20 percent maximum.* There are no "good fats" (other than an omega-3 supplement). Coconut oil and olive oil is not "good for you"—no matter what you read somewhere. All trans-fats and hydrogenated fats and oils have to be totally avoided. Just read your labels. Labels that read "Trans-Fat Free" can still contain some under the FDA rules. Red meats, such as beef, pork, and lamb, are too full of saturated fat and cholesterol to be good food choices. The ideal is to give up meat completely. Just bite the bullet and give up meat! You don't need it, and you aren't meant to eat it.

- **Poultry and eggs** are among the top ten allergenic foods, along with milk and dairy products. Chicken, turkey, duck, quail, goose, pigeon, and pheasant are all the same basically. One large egg has a whopping 250 mg of artery clogging cholesterol. Eating egg whites or egg substitutes is not the answer here either. Just take poultry and eggs out of your diet. Eat turkey on Thanksgiving and Christmas every year if you wish.

DASH Diet

The DASH Diet must be mentioned again. Yes, this diet is a step in the right direction, and certainly easier for people to adapt to than macrobiotics. Whole grains are emphasized as your major food. Vegetables are emphasized as your secondary food. The promoters have no idea that Nightshade foods should be avoided. They also don't understand that tropical vegetables are meant only for tropical people in tropical climates. Fruits are recommended as your third-most important food, when you don't need any fruit at all. Fruit should be limited to 10 percent of your daily food intake. They advise 4 to 5 servings a day. They also advise 2 to 3 servings of dairy products. *You should have zero dairy foods in your life.* They suggest only 2 or fewer servings a day of meat, poultry, or fish. One serving of fish would be even better. Most people simply do not want to give up meat, poultry, eggs, or dairy. Beans, legumes, nuts, and seeds are recommended less than one serving a day! *Beans and legumes should be eaten every day, and are a major staple second only to whole grains.* You certainly don't want to limit them to less than a serving a day. All in all, they suggest you eat a whopping 19 to 24 servings of food a day! You only need two small meals a day, or about 8 servings. One reason Americans are so sickly is that they eat twice the calories they need. Men only need about 1,800 calories, and women only about 1,200 calories. The DASH Diet just doesn't go far enough at all, but it is certainly in the right direction.

Terry Shintani (*American Journal of Clinical Nutrition* v 53, 1991) fed obese, sickly native Hawaiians all the natural food they wanted for a mere three weeks. These were low-fat, high-fiber, low-protein meals of taro, poi, yams, breadfruit, fruits, fish, and other traditional foods. They didn't even exercise! *Their health changed completely in only 21 days,* and their blood pressures fell 11.5 mm (systolic) and 8.9 mm (diastolic). That's dramatic! Dr. Shintani is a very sincere man and author of two good books.

At Deakin University, men ate the DASH Diet for 12 weeks. Their baseline pressures were 129 and 81, and dropped to 124 and 76. Their body weight fell as well, by a whopping 12 pounds just by eating healthier foods. At the University of Calgary they got even better results with the DASH Diet with a reduction of 11.4 and 5.5 mm in systolic and diastolic pressures, in only 60 days. Obese hypertensives at the University of South Carolina went on the DASH Diet and got very impressive reductions of 8.1 and 7.4 mm in their pressures in only 4 weeks. At the University of Tehran 116 patients went on the DASH Diet for six months. Their HDL went up, and their LDL went down, along with total cholesterol, systolic (11 mm) and diastolic pressures (7 mm), blood sugar, and body weight. The most comprehensive review was from Boston University listing the various DASH studies. Yes, this works and proves better food choices lower blood pressure. Admittedly, this is a more appealing approach to the masses, since they can include some meat and dairy, and eat lots of calories. It just doesn't go far enough.

The Mediterranean Diet will also lower blood pressure somewhat, but this has many problems. Meat and dairy, especially cheese, are included. Most of the rice, pasta and bread are white, rather than whole grain. Nightshades, especially tomatoes, are daily vegetables for this diet. The Mediterranean Diet just isn't any good.

The best choices of all are the rural Asian diets in general—China, Japan, Thailand, Viet Nam. Rural Asians overall are the healthiest people in the world. The rural Japanese and Okinawans are the best examples. Urban Asians have adopted too many Western dietary habits overall.

Other Diets

Fad diets come and go like subway trains. There is always a new Magic Diet for the great unwashed masses. Since they don't work, they eventually fade away. This includes the Zone Diet, the Atkins Diet, the South Beach Diet, the Blood Type Diet, and the Glycemic Index. However, some have survived. Jenny Craig and Weight Watchers keep rolling along no matter how ineffective they are.

Now we have the irrational Gluten-Free Diet and the Paleo Diet. The Ketogenic Diet keeps reincarnating under different names like the Evolution Diet. The diet books in print are generally of very poor quality, to say the least. Unfortunately macrobiotics is not well known anymore. This is a shame. People are just not willing to stop eating meat, poultry, eggs, dairy foods, refined foods, sugar, and desserts. It is sad that the most powerful diet regimen ever known is fading into obscurity.

George Ohsawa wrote some very brief and simple books on the basic Japanese oriented diet, as did Michio Kushi, Herman

Aihara, and other macrobiotic authors. All this was far too Japan oriented, too restricted, and too limited though.

None of the above authors, unfortunately, know anything about proven supplements, natural hormone balance, and fasting. Nor do they stress exercise. Real macrobiotics (overall view of life) should be about life extension and ultimate health. This must include proven supplements, natural hormone balance, regular exercise, and weekly fasting. Read the *Seven Steps* on page 119 at the end of this book.

CALORIE RESTRICTIONS

Calorie restriction is an important part of macrobiotics and life extension. *Eat as little as possible by choosing low calorie foods.* Eat as few calories as possible by making better food choices, *not* by going hungry! You can eat fewer calories by choosing whole grains, beans, most vegetables, local fruits, good soups, good salads, and seafood. Americans eat twice the calories they need. *A man only needs about 1,800 calories a day, and a woman only about 1,200.* Just eat two meals a day; you don't need three.

Roy Walford is the only one who wrote extensively on the subject of calorie restriction. *The 120-Year Diet* and *Maximum Lifespan* are his best. Science has verified the power of long-term caloric restriction in monkeys and higher primates, and short term in humans. *Calorie restriction is the single most effective method to prolong life.* You do this by making better food choices. You take in fewer calories by eating all the low fat natural foods you want, not by going hungry. Eat two meals a day, take your lunch to work, don't eat out often, fast once a week, do a two day fast once a month. *Just make better food choices,* and you can eat all you want. Whole, low-fat foods are the key here.

FASTING

Fasting one day a week from dinner to dinner is another way to eat less. A two day fast every month adds to this. Don't think that you can't go a mere 24 hours on water. You'll find the one day fast completely effortless after a few months. You will actually come to looking forward to your one day weekly fast, since you'll feel much lighter and better with no food in your stomach. Short-term fasting is actually pleasurable. Longer-term fasting is more arduous, but also far more rewarding. Authors who have written good fasting books include Paul and Patricia Bragg, Alan Cott, Lee Bueno, Dave Williams, Norbert Kriegisch, and Eve Adamson.

CONCLUSION

You can lower your blood pressure with diet and lifestyle, rather than toxic drugs. This chapter has outlined the foods to include in your diet to cure your hypertension, and the foods to be eliminated. The next chapter addresses obesity, an epidemic in the U.S., and its negative effect on your health, including the higher risk for getting serious diseases.

6. Obesity Is Basic

America is the fattest nation on earth, and it is literally getting fatter every day. We eat twice the calories we need, twice the protein we need, eight times the fat we need, and 160 pounds of sugars we don't have any need for. We are the most affluent nation on earth, with the highest standard of living. This combination always brings poor health and high rates of disorders, such as cancer, diabetes, and heart disease. Obesity is linked to higher rates of every medical condition known. (The exception is osteoporosis, since the bones must be stronger to support all the extra weight.)

One-third of American adults are obese, and many of the rest are overweight. Nearly all Americans are out of shape, and get no real exercise. *Eighty percent of diabetics are obese.* One in three American children today will grow up diabetic! Obesity is second only to diet in causing hypertension. We have to keep going back to the fact that high blood pressure is mainly due to insulin resistance. Insulin resistance is, in fact, prediabetes. All of these factors are just aspects of the same basic blood sugar dysmetabolism.

WEIGHT LOSS AIDS

No diet aid works. There are no magic weight loss supplements, and never will be. There are no chemical shortcuts. None of the diet supplements or drugs work. Bariatric surgery isn't the answer, and it will destroy your health. If any of these methods worked, then obesity would be cured, and would be obsolete. You don't lose weight with magic supplements. You lose weight with diet and lifestyle, by making better food choices. Dean Ornish's book *Eat More, Weigh Less* is a good example of this. Terri Shintani's books *The Hawaii Diet* and *The Good Carbohydrate Revolution* are other fine books.

RESEARCH RELATING OBESITY TO HYPERTENSION

The harmfulness of being overweight is agreed upon literally by every scientist in the world. Let's take a quick look at some of the best of the countless studies about obesity.

The University of Valencia in Spain said the association between obesity and hypertension has been well documented in most all racial, ethnic, and socio-economic groups. They suggested long term dietary treatment, and reducing calorie intake through better diet, instead of the usual drug regimen.

At the Jiangxi Hospital in China they concluded that the BMI (body mass index) has a close correlation with blood pressure and serum lipid level. Hypertension increases dramatically in women after menopause, largely due to the increased hormone imbalance, not lower estradiol and estrone levels. Low range estrogen levels are actually the ideal. Low progesterone is another factor.

At McMaster University in Canada they claimed that the relationship between obesity, hypertension, and insulin resistance is well recognized.

At Sahigrenska Hospital in Sweden they concluded that their findings suggest that general and central obesity is independently related to blood pressure.

Human clinical studies done at the famous Cornell University (*American Journal of Clinical Nutrition* v 46, 1987) demonstrated that you can eat all you want and never be hungry. Women were allowed to eat all they wanted 24 hours a day nonstop, as long as they ate the offered healthy natural foods. All of these had 20 percent or less fat calories. A control group was allowed 30 percent fat-calorie foods. It really is very easy to limit your fat intake to one-fifth of your calories. The first group of women had impressive weight loss in just 30 days, while eating all they wanted 24 hours a day. The second group lost no weight at all. Again, the average American chugs down 42 percent fat, which is nearly all saturated, artery clogging animal fat from meat, poultry, eggs, and dairy. This is just one of many published studies proving that food per se doesn't make you fat—*it's fat that makes you fat*. This is a wonderful study.

WHAT TO EAT AND HOW MUCH?

Eat low-fat, high-fiber natural foods, such as whole grains, beans, vegetables, fruits, seafood, soups, and salads. As shown in the research conducted at Cornell University, *you can eat all you want and never be hungry. The magic number here is 20 percent or less fat calories.* If you eat, say, 8 ounces of salmon at 30 percent fat you must balance this with 8 ounces of brown rice or 8 ounces of cooked beans. Just 14 ounces of peanuts, or 19 ounces of sirloin steak, have 2,500 calories, most all of them from fat. That's far more than a grown man needs in a whole day. On the other hand, you would need to eat over five pounds of brown rice, over five pounds of pinto beans, or six pounds of cooked oatmeal to get the same amount of calories.

Since everyone is in agreement about obesity being a major cause of blood pressure problems, the question really is how can we stay slim and healthy without being hungry? *By making better food choices.* It really is that simple . . . make better food choices. That's how. You can eat all you want, never be hungry, and stay slim and healthy all your life. Just choose healthier foods to eat. The basic thing to understand is that food doesn't make you fat; *it's fat that makes you fat.* Carbohydrates and protein contain only 5 calories per gram, while fat contains a whopping 9 calories. We're going to purposely review some things from Chapter 5: Diet, Diet, Diet for added emphasis.

The first food group to go is milk and dairy products of all kinds, even the low-fat and no-fat ones. All dairy foods contain indigestible allergenic lactose (milk sugar). All adults of all races are allergic to lactose, as they no longer secrete the enzyme lactase. Dairy foods also contain the cancer promoting amino acid casein. It is easier than you think to drop the dairy habit, and stop listening to ads that say, "Got milk?" Soy, rice, almond milk, and other milks are very tasty, and readily available in mainstream grocery chains from various makers in a variety of flavors. You'll come to prefer them over dairy.

Beef, pork, lamb, and other red meats need to be eliminated. Meat is full of saturated fat, animal proteins, cholesterol, and calories. People addicted to meat can at least limit this to one lean four ounce serving a day. Yes, red meat is an addiction for many. However, you'll never be healthy, even when eating small amounts of meat.

Poultry and eggs also must be omitted. Poultry (of all kinds) and eggs are two of the most allergenic of all foods. Many people have unrecognized allergies to them. Poultry is full of fat, cholesterol, and animal protein. A single egg has a whopping 250 mg of artery clogging cholesterol; two eggs have 500 mg. Eating only egg whites is not the answer at all.

Americans eat a mere 1 percent of whole grains. At least half your diet should be comprised of whole grains. *Whole grains are the staff of life, your main staple, the very basis of your daily fare.* Replace white rice with brown, white bread and white pasta with 100 percent whole grain. Eat hot and cold 100 percent whole grain breakfast cereals. Get a good cookbook that emphasizes whole grain recipes.

OTHER FACTORS AFFECTING YOUR WEIGHT

Hormones have a strong influence on weight , BMI, and percent body fat. Almost everyone over the age of 40 has some kind of hormone imbalance, as well as some people under 40. DHEA, testosterone estradiol, estrone, T3, and T4 are especially important for weight management.

Proven supplements keep your **metabolism** at peak performance. People over 40 should be taking acidophilus, beta-sitosterol, beta glucan, beta-carotene, CoQ10, DIM, flax oil, FOS, glutamine, glucosamine, lipoic acid, sulforaphane, minerals and vitamins, NAC, PS, quercetin, soy isoflavones, vitamin D, and vitamin E.

The importance of **exercise** for weight management cannot be overemphasized. You can lose weight simply by taking a half hour brisk walk every day.

Weekly **fasting** can be a great way to maintain your weight. Just fast on water from dinner to dinner one day a week. You can also add a two day monthly fast.

Never take **prescription drugs** as they imbalance your system. Americans take more prescription drugs by far than anyone else on earth. You'll never be healthy or happy while poisoning yourself with synthetic, toxic prescription chemicals. You can't drug yourself to health. Drugs just cover up the symptoms, while making your health worse.

Stop any **bad habits**, like coffee. Bad habits breed bad habits, and just encourage you to overeat. Success breeds success. Failure breeds failure.

CONCLUSION

Obesity doesn't just cause high blood pressure and cardiovascular disease. *Obesity is closely correlated to every known medical condition and illness. Obesity is a direct cause of all-cause mortality.* Overweight people die early and have a poor quality of life.

The Birmingham Factory Screening Project was one of countless such studies to prove this. Here 2,878 English adults were studied and closely monitored for a full 18 years. This was a costly and rare ongoing study. "In conclusion obesity is a significant influence on blood pressure and all-cause mortality in this large cohort of subjects screened and followed up for 18 years."

7. The Minerals You Need

Every disease and known health condition is due in part to mineral deficiency. You are simply not going to get well until you get all the known minerals you need. There are at least 24 known elements we need, and we get enough sodium, potassium, phosphorous, and sulfur in our diets. Yet, there are only ten elements classified scientifically as essential. We know there are more than twice that many. *All Your Minerals*® was developed with 20 elements in the amounts you need. The FDA then banned all use of germanium, cesium, and gallium. That still leaves 17, and this is the best mineral supplement available by far.

In the last twenty years of international published research there are two studies that stand out. Hubert Loyke, at St. Vincents Hospital in Cleveland, wrote extensive articles (*Biological Trace Element Research* v 58, 1997 and v. 85, 2002). He discussed 28 different elements and their effect on blood pressure. At the Medical University in Lodz, 23 elements were studied in humans with hypertension (*Klinika Kardiologica* v 8, 2004). In Russia at the Institute of Earth Crust, 23 elements were studied in patients with high blood pressure (*Nutrition* v 11, 1995). All of these were very clear about the importance of getting the minerals we need to maintain normal blood pressure. Research like this is priceless, and shows the real cure for any illness is to treat the cause with nutrition, rather than cover it up with toxic chemicals. At the University of Manitoba (*Nutritional Research Reviews* v 14, 2001) using minerals and vitamins to lower blood pressure was studied, rather than harmful drugs. Doctors like these deserve a lot of credit. Nehru University in New Delhi also showed that minerals are the way to treat hypertension rather than drugs (*Biological Trace Element Research* v 34, 1992).

The real point, which will be repeated over and over, is that we need all the known minerals, not just some of them. Magnesium, calcium, zinc, copper, chromium, selenium, and vanadium have been studied more than any other elements, but it is almost impossible to do studies on the ultratrace minerals since their effects are so subtle.

VITAL MINERALS

We need to realize that we need *all* the vital minerals our bodies require, and not just the most "important." *Minerals work together as a team in harmony and synergy with each other.* The ideal way to get the minerals we need is to take a supplement with all 17 of the ones we know we need. Let's look in detail at the specific elements:

Boron

Boron is probably *the most deficient mineral in our diet.* There is no official RDA, but 3 mg is the suggested daily intake. It wasn't until 1990 that boron was even accepted as essential! The research is overwhelming here. Our soils and food are very boron deficient. You would think all vitamin and mineral supplements would contain 3 mg of this inexpensive and vital element, but many do not. This proves the megacorporations have huge advertising budgets but no research departments. Americans probably only take in a mere 1 mg a day. Be sure you get this in your supplement, as boron deficiency is all too common. Citrates or common boric acid are beneficial.

Calcium

Calcium has a lot of research for blood pressure. This emphasis on calcium is misleading, however, as are the amounts recommended. Europeans in all countries (along with India) have the highest calcium intake in the world from all the dairy products they consume. Be clear that *there is very little calcium in any food group other than dairy products.* The only high calcium foods are dairy products, and no one should be eating milk and milk products. Americans and Europeans also have the highest blood pressure, along with the Japanese.

The official RDA of 1,000 mg a day is simply ridiculous, clinically unsupported, and completely contradicted by epidemiological studies of billions of people. *A realistic intake would be 250 mg* from your diet. This is about what billions of Asians and Africans take in every day. You could possibly add another 250 mg from supplementation. The usual citrates and carbonates are effective. There is just no reason at all to overdose on calcium. *The RDA is simply wrong. If Nature wanted us to eat more calcium, it would not be limited to dairy foods.*

At the Department of Public Health in Japan (*Maguneshumu* v. 10, 1991) *hypertension patients were shown to actually have higher blood calcium levels.* Healthy Pima Indians were shown (*Journal of the American College of Nutrition* v. 17, 1998) to have lower blood pressure along with lower blood calcium than normal. The real problem with calcium is not intake at all but rather *absorption.* You need magnesium, boron, silicon, strontium, vitamin D, testosterone, progesterone, and omega-3 fatty acids, among other nutrients, to properly absorb the calcium you eat.

Cesium

Cesium is an important ultratrace mineral, and 100 mcg is all you need. Do not take more than that. Human blood, common food, and soil studies prove how vital this is for our health. You won't find it in mineral supplements since it was banned by the FDA in 2015. International studies show the importance of cesium in our soil, our food, and our blood. Cesium is vital for humans and animals. Soon science will admit this and set an RDA. Regular salts, especially chloride, work well here.

Chromium

Chromium only recently has an RDA of 120 mcg. This is often deficient in our diet, due to the refining of the grains we eat. It is critical for proper blood sugar metabolism, and deficiency is one of the reasons for such an epidemic. Never exceed an intake of more than 400 mcg. This has a very low toxicity. Regular chelates (a non-metal ion bound to a metal ion for better absorbability) are the best sources, not patented forms.

Cobalt

Cobalt is almost never found in mineral supplements, even though it is the basic building block for vitamin B-12. Food and blood studies prove its importance. We synthesize our own B-12, but we cannot do this without cobalt in our blood. We probably only take in about 25 mcg or less, but that is enough. This may not sound like much, but we only need to make about 3 mcg of B-12 daily. Taking B-12 orally just doesn't work, so you must take 1 mg of methyl cobalamin. It must be emphasized that sufficient B-12 is just not found in foods, is orally unavailable, and that a cobalt supplement should insure that you synthesize the 3 mcg you need every day. Remember that regular B-12 is not orally available.

Copper

Copper also has an RDA of only 2 mg. Americans probably only take in about half this amount. Some people with hypertension have excessive levels, while others are deficient. Whole grains and beans are the best source. Our bodies only contain a total of about 150 mg of this vital element. That's all. Taking 2 mg in your supplement is good insurance. It would take about 15 mg a day for toxicity, which is very unlikely. Citrates, oxides, and gluconates are all very well absorbed.

Gallium

Gallium is definitely a required ultratrace element, and 100 mcg is all you need. The earth's crust has an amazing 10 mg per kg of this vital element. Human blood has shown about 30 pcg per 100 ml. It is found in most all common foods. Seafood has about 0.15 mg per kg. It is especially important for bone metabolism. Estimates are that we only take in about 12 mcg. Nitrate is a good form. Any use of gallium was irrationally banned by the FDA in 2015.

Germanium

Germanium is a very important ultratrace element that was banned by the FDA in 2015. You only need about 100 mcg of ultratrace elements like germanium. Do not exceed this amount, however, as 100 mcg is sufficient. Clinical human blood studies prove this is a vital element we need, but our soils and our food are deficient, and it is not found in supplements. Germanium sesquoxide and chelates are safe, but germanium dioxide is not. Any use of germanium was irrationally banned by the FDA.

Iodine

Iodine is very important, and the only other nonmetallic element we need to supplement. The RDA is a mere 150 mcg. Eating sea vegetables like kelp, nori, and hijiki regularly, as many Asians do, is not a good idea surprisingly. All seaweed contains extreme amounts of iodine. Kombu, for example, contains a massive 250 mg (not mcg) per 100 g. Overdoses of any mineral unbalance your metabolism, and are not simply excreted without effect. The most important value here is thyroid metabolism. There are only about 30 mg in our bodies, and three-fourths of this is in our thyroid gland. Only 30 mg. Iodine supplements, however, will just not correct any thyroid problems. You need actual thyroid hormones T3 and T4 to do that.

Iron

Iron deficiency is as common as ever. High levels of iron are rarely found in hypertension. High blood levels of iron is due to an excretion problem, and not excessive intake. Iron retention, and lack of excretion, is a rather rare problem. Iron is the "heme" in hemoglobin, and the basic mineral in our blood. A good supplement will contain the female RDA of 18 mg. The male RDA is only 10 mg. Common sulfates, fumarates, and gluconates are good choices.

Magnesium

Magnesium deficiency is very common since we eat so few whole grains. Plants use magnesium as the core for chlorophyll, as mammals use iron as the core for blood. Eating a whole grain based diet should give you about 400 mg a day, and you can add a supplement of at least 200 mg. Over dosing on magnesium, or any other mineral, is not the answer here at all. The average American probably only gets about 300 mg a day due to the heavily refined foods they eat. Studies show that one in seven Americans is seriously deficient in blood magnesium. The best source of all is whole grains, *but we eat a mere one percent whole grains in our diet. If you eat whole grains, you really don't need a supplement. Study after study shows low blood magnesium in hypertension patients. Citrates, lactates, and oxides are effective.*

Manganese

Manganese is very important, and the RDA was only recently established at 2 mg. Whole grains are a major source, along with beans, legumes, nuts, and some vegetables. There is an abundance of research about the benefits for our health. A 2 mg supplement is good insurance for such an important element. We only have a total of about 20 mg of manganese in our bodies. That's all, 20 mg. Whole grains, beans, and leafy green vegetables are the best sources. Sulfates and oxides are effective.

Molybdenum

Molybdenum has an RDA of 75 mcg, but that may not be enough. Be sure to take a supplement here to insure adequate intake. All common salts are good sources, and you will find this in all your supplement formulas. Molybdenum is safe and non-toxic, even though it is a heavy metal. The research is concerned more with soil and plants, rather than animals and humans. Farmers and gardeners commonly use this in their fertilizer and animal feed.

Nickel

Nickel is an ignored ultratrace element; 100 mcg is all you need. Food and blood analysis of animals and humans show this is an essential element, but there is little research on its benefits, or on the problems caused by deficiency. The research is mostly for soil and crops. Nickel is needed in human and animal nutrition. You won't find this in the mineral supplements on the market either—except All Your Minerals®. Regular salts, such as chlorides and sulfates, are good.

Rubidium

Rubidium is not an ultratrace element at all, as our intake is about 1 mg (1,000 mcg). Taking a supplement of 500 mcg is enough, since common rubidium deficiency has not been demonstrated. This is never found in mineral supplements (except one), and very ignored by science. Found abundantly in soil and crops, as well as in animals and humans. The few studies we have are very positive. This is definitely required in human, animal, and plant nutrition. Rubidium is found in fruits, vegetables, poultry, and seafood. Chloride is a good form to use.

Selenium

Selenium finally has an official RDA of 70 mcg, but it was ignored until very recently. It is very deficient in both our soils and heavily refined foods. Do not exceed a daily intake of more than 200 mcg, as this is a heavy metal and will accumulate in your body.

Whole grains are the very best source. Chelates are the most absorbable form of selenium. Studies show that people with low blood selenium suffer from higher disease rates, such as cancer, coronary heart disease, and diabetes.

Silicon

Silicon is the ignored or "orphan mineral," and almost never found in mineral supplements. There is no RDA set for this, but 10 mg a day is a safe and effective dose. Do not use horsetail as a source. Silica levels in our foods vary so greatly, that it is all but impossible to say which foods are good sources. Bone and joint health depend on silica as a basic building block. The science here is most impressive. Plain silica gel (silicic acid) is a good and inexpensive source. You aren't going to find this in the vast majority of mineral supplements; it is in *All Your Minerals*® of course. This is one of the two nonmetallic elements we need.

Strontium

Strontium is another very important trace element with very good science behind it. You will rarely find it in mineral supplements, but 1 mg (1,000 mcg) is a good dose. Bone and joint health depend on strontium as a building block, as does calcium absorption. No RDA has been set, but science finally recognizes this as essential. Do not confuse it with the radioactive form strontium-90. Chelates and asparates are good choices.

Tin

Tin is also ignored as a necessary ultratrace element; 100 mcg is a good dose. Common food and soil studies prove this is an essential element. Most of the research has been concerned with tin toxicity from industrial pollution, instead of the benefits. Unfortunately, the FDA irrationally limits the dose to 30 mcg. You never find tin in mineral supplements, except one. Human studies have shown low blood tin levels in some illnesses, so we need more research here. Regular salts, such as chlorides and sulfates, are well absorbed.

Vanadium

Vanadium was ignored until very recently, and still there is no RDA for it. It is now officially accepted as essential. Taking 1 mg (1,000 mcg) a day is good, but almost no supplements contain this vital mineral. Do not exceed 2 mg a day, as this is toxic at 10 mg. Very low toxicity ceiling. Vanadium has been shown to be critical for blood sugar metabolism. Deficiency is all too common, due to our intake of refined foods. There is now very good science on the importance of vanadium, especially for blood pressure and blood sugar dysmetabolism. Chelates and sulfates are your best choices here.

Zinc

Zinc may be either high or low in those with hypertension; there is just no consistency here. Most people do not get the 15 mg RDA they need from the food they eat. Zinc is found in whole grains, beans, nuts, and meats. Deficiency is especially true for the poor, elderly, and alcoholics. There are about 2.5 g of zinc in the human body, half of which is in the muscles. Whole grains and beans are the best sources. *Never take in more than 50 mg of zinc daily.* The toxicity level is very low. The usual citrates, oxides, and sulfates all work well.

What about Potassium?

We get plenty of this in our diets. The National Institute of Health in Framingham showed serum potassium is not related to blood pressure (*American Journal of Hypertension* v 15, 2002) with thousands of patients. Almost no studies find any benefits for potassium supplements.

Other Ultratrace Elements

In the future, we will find other ultratrace elements are also vital for our health and well-being. It is *very* difficult to study these ultratrace elements, since they occur in such tiny microgram amounts in our food and in our bodies.

Barium is essential.

Cerium is found in humans and animals.

Colloidal silver is a scam, and there is no evidence that silver is needed in human nutrition.

Europium may well be essential, and science will probably decide this in the next decade.

Indium is claimed to be effective, but studies do not support the Internet ads you see for it.

Lanthanum has considerable research, and it is probably vital.

Lithium is essential, but we probably get enough in our daily food. (Megadoses of lithium for depression is medical insanity.)

Neodymium has shown promise in both animal and human studies.

Praseodymium has some animal and human nutrition research to indicate possible importance.

Scandium is proven to be a necessary nutrient.

Thulium (not thallium) has also shown promise, but only in soil and plant studies so far.

Titanium is essential.

Tungsten is definitely required in human nutrition.

There are other ultratrace elements that may also be found to be vital. Meanwhile, if you eat whole natural foods and take the seventeen elements we need, you'll be fine. Look on the Internet and Google "mineral supplements."

"BAD" MINERALS

While these good minerals support our health, the "bad" minerals do the opposite. Due to industrial pollution, there are elements that build up in our systems, raise our blood pressure, and cause other problems. These include, lead, cadmium, aluminum, arsenic, mercury, and thallium.

Lead *is the most prominent toxic metal for humans* (especially for African Americans, but not Africans), with aluminum second. Mercury and cadmium are lesser common toxins, along with arsenic and thallium.

The Burns and Allen Research Institute in Los Angeles did an entire study (*Medical Hypotheses* v 59, 2002) showing how common lead toxicity is, and that it is a significant cause of high blood pressure. It is a good idea to get a blood (not hair or urine) test for these toxic metals.

Aluminum is the only lightweight toxic element. Alzheimer's is strongly correlated with high blood and brain aluminum levels. Do not use regular baking powder (use sodium based instead), or deodorants with aluminum salts (98 percent of commercial deodorants).

Eating well, calorie restriction, exercise, and weekly fasting are good ways to lower these toxic metals. Three grams daily of sodium alginate, a seaweed extract, for six to twelve months is a good way to get these metals out of your body. (Just Google "sodium alginate" on the Internet for a source.)

CONCLUSION

We are all mineral deficient, no matter how well we eat, and very few people eat well at all. One of the basic causes of hypertension and blood sugar dysmetabolism is mineral deficiency. Research cited in this chapter is priceless, and shows that the real cure for any illness is to treat the cause with nutrition, rather than harmful drugs. Now you know the minerals necessary to maintain a healthy blood pressure level, the next chapter covers the myths of low sodium diets.

8. The Low Sodium Myth

You *do not need to go on a low sodium diet.* This is the most pervasive myth about curing high blood pressure. This is a real urban legend. The word "salary" comes from the Latin word for salt, "sal." Roman soldiers were paid in part with salt, because of its great value. Salt has been used as currency throughout human history. You'll find the word salt throughout the Bible. We're all familiar with phrases such as, "salt of the earth." Animals naturally gravitate towards a salt block to lick it.

That is not to say, however, that you can eat all the added salt you want. You do, however, have to moderate your salt intake. There are far too many citations to list on this. The average American is estimated to eat almost nine grams of salt daily. Six grams would be much more reasonable. You simply need to *moderate* the salt in your daily food. Whole grains, beans, vegetables, fruits, and seafood have little sodium. Even beef, pork, poultry, and eggs have less than 100 mg of sodium, generally, per (3.5 ounce) serving. *Ninety percent of your sodium intake comes from sodium chloride added to your food.* Processing and salt shakers are the only two real sources.

THE LOW SODIUM MYTH

There are many pseudoarguments for the low sodium myth. For example, there is a popular argument that some primitive cultures have a low salt intake along with an absence of hypertension.

When they adopt the Western diet, and double their salt intake, they sometimes suffer from high blood pressure. The problem here is that *their entire diet and lifestyle changes!* You can't single out salt when their entire diet and way of life changes completely. There are too many variables to even count in such a situation.

Salt intake, basically, does not equate to blood pressure, except in people with kidney conditions who are also "salt-sensitive." *Decreasing salt intake does not lower blood pressure.* The average American probably takes in about 9 grams of sodium chloride. This comes from processing and your salt shaker. Peanuts, for example, only have 5 mg of sodium per (3.5 oz) serving, but peanut butter has over 600 mg! Pork has only about 65 mg per serving, but pork sausage a whopping 1,000 mg! Pickles of various kinds, olives, salted nuts, chips, and popcorn have extreme amounts of salt in them. Such foods can only be eaten in moderation, or better, just avoided.

Again, this is not to say you can just eat all the salt and salted foods you want. Common sense tells you that. Our kidneys regulate the sodium level in our blood, and excrete the excess. High salt intake stresses, overworks, and eventually wears out the kidneys. Kidney disease is epidemic in the West generally, but *this is due to excess protein intake,* not sodium. The best blood tests for this are creatinine and albumin. Increased overall mortality has also been correlated with eating too much salt. High salt intake has clearly been shown to reduce insulin sensitivity as well. *Moderation in everything.* You should not eat an excessive amount of any food, obviously, and that certainly includes salt.

The Japanese eat more salt than anyone on earth. One

problem with the traditional Japanese macrobiotic diet is the high salt intake; pickled vegetables, salt-pressed salad, daily miso soup, high-sodium tamari soy sauce, gomasio, and natto as condiments. It all adds up to a salt overload.

THE RESEARCH

The famous Framingham Study proved this beyond any doubt. Salt intake was proven to be unrelated to hypertension (except for people with serious kidney conditions). The Framingham Study is the longest, largest, ongoing study on cardiovascular health ever done. Studies, such as the fine, double-blind one done at the University of Barcelona (*Clinical Science* v 101, 2001), simply could not raise blood pressure in people consuming large amounts of added salt.

It should be mentioned that black people, and other ethnic groups, are far more salt-sensitive, and prone to hypertension. They must moderate their salt intake (*Journal of the American College of Nutrition* v 14, 1995). This study also showed that only a few salt-sensitive people, with weakened kidney function, benefited from low salt diets. Other misleading, "salt is bad for you" studies find irrelevant changes in blood pressure (for example, 128 mm instead of 130 mm), yet claim significant changes due to low salt intake.

An 11 page study (*Medical Hypotheses* v 63, 2004) with a full 145 references, was very clear about this. If sodium alone raised blood pressure, why don't common sodium salts like citrate and bicarbonate do the same? *They don't.* If sodium was the problem, any edible sodium compound would act just the same as sodium chloride. Again, about 90 percent of our sodium intake comes from the salt shaker and the processed foods we eat. *Food itself contains very little sodium.*

On the other hand, severely restricting salt intake can actually cause problems, like excessive renin, high angiotensin levels, and sympathetic activity. At the University of Milan (*Circulation* v 106, 2002) hypertensives were given a severely restricted salt diet. The doctors found, "A moderate dietary Na (sodium chloride) restriction triggers a sympathetic activation and a baroflex impairment. Maintenance of the low-Na diet for several weeks does not attenuate these adverse adrenergic and reflex effects." In plain words *you need a little added salt in your diet.* Moderation in all things.

Salt Intake And High Blood Pressure

Aren't there published studies to prove salt intake raises blood pressure? Well, the closer you look at these studies, the less you see. At Catholic University in South Korea (*Electrolyte & Blood Pressure* v 3, 2005) the doctors made this claim. The actual results showed a very slight fall of 1.5 mm in diastolic pressure when people who used excessive salt were put on a low-salt diet. This is not a relevant figure.

At the famous Johns Hopkins University (*American Journal of Clinical Nutrition* v 65, 1997), they got a mere 1.2 mm reduction in diastolic pressure by severely restricting salt. They found that weight loss did, in fact, lower their pressures substantially.

At Hirosaki University in Japan (*Blood Purification* v 20, 2002) doctors compared two groups of people. One group ate just 2 grams of salt a day, while the second group ate over 21 grams! Such obviously faulty studies like this are prima facie meaningless. Other studies put the patients on better diets and had them exercise. Then they attributed any improvement in blood pressure solely to salt restriction: Junk science.

It is salt-sensitive people, with chronic kidney weakness, who are affected by added salt. This is due to poor kidney function, rather than salt intake. Doctors at St. George's Hospital in London (*Hypertension* v 45, 2004) were very clear about this. ". . .those who develop high blood pressure have an underlying defect in the ability of the kidney to excrete salt." Japanese doctors (*Nippon Kaisui* v 59, 2005) said, "Salt restriction is only effective in salt-sensitive subjects. Strict salt restriction might be of hazard to health. The policy of universal salt restriction should be avoided." *The real issue with kidneys is protein intake,* not just added salt. Americans eat twice the protein they need, which damages the kidneys, raises blood urea, and causes a whole host of health problems. A macrobiotic diet is very low in protein, and only includes 10 percent fish and seafood at most. It is very important to stop eating red meat, poultry, dairy, and eggs due to the high protein content, as well as the high fat content of these foods. High protein diets will kill you. Some people are just incapable of taking animal foods out of their life.

The real cause of hypertension, more than anything else is various sugars and sugar substitutes, not salt. Eating sugar raises insulin levels, which in turn, causes salt reabsorption, rather than excretion (*Rinsho Byori* v 55, 2007). Our completely irresponsible intake of 160 pounds of various simple sugars every year is the major cause of blood sugar disorders, and resultant high blood pressure.

Are Potassium Supplements Needed In Our Diet?

What about potassium, since there is a vital potassium to sodium balance in our bodies maintained by our kidneys? Potassium supplements rarely have any benefit, and potassium is sufficient in our food.

Doctors at St. George's Hospital (*Hypertension* v 45, 2005) just got no benefit from giving people 2,300 mg potassium supplements. Even large doses like this just have no value. The best potassium source is various fruits. Still, you should limit fruit intake to 10 percent of your diet or less. *You really don't even need to eat any fruit, since it is so low in nutrition.* Cooked beans have very high potassium levels of 400 to 500 mg a cup. Cooked brown rice, for example, has about 137 mg per cup. Men take in about 3,000 mg of potassium a day, and women about 2,400 mg a day.

What about the salt substitutes made of both sodium and potassium chlorides? They are expensive, taste metallic, and are just not necessary. In Brazil (*Revista de Nutricao* v 18, 2005) such substitutes were given to people with no benefit at all.

CONCLUSION

The low-sodium diet is a myth. *Simply moderate your salt intake, and lower your protein intake.* Moderate the salt you add to your food. Avoid salted snacks, pickles, and olives. Read the labels on all processed foods, their sodium content. Salt in moderation is necessary for life.

9. The Supplements You Need

Supplements are very powerful and effective, but *only* if you are eating and living well. If you are not eating a good whole grain based low-fat diet, no amount of supplements is going to help you very much. If you are under 40, you should not have high blood pressure in the first place. Those under 40 only need about eight supplements. These are beta glucan, a mineral supplement, a vitamin supplement, vitamin E, vitamin D, FOS, acidophilus, and flax oil. L-glutamine can be added to that list. Most of the following supplements are not directly related to blood pressure, but they are vital for overall health. Treat your whole body, and not merely the dual pressures of your blood. *Holistic health treats the entire body as a whole,* not just one organ or one condition. The healthier your entire body is, the healthier your cardiovascular system will be.

If you are over 40, you should be taking about 18 proven supplements, plus any hormones you need. If you don't see a certain supplement mentioned here it is because it is exogenous (temporary), or there is no science behind it, despite its popularity. Lycopene, poliosanol, resveratrol, chondroitin, homeopathic remedies, 5-HTP, spirulina, maca, saw palmetto, MSM, oral SOD, acai, and other such products simply have no published, human, clinical supporting science.

PROVEN SUPPLEMENTS TO TAKE

Acetyl-l-carnitine (ALC) is simply a more effective form of the amino acid l-carnitine, and is more absorbable. Take 500 mg a day. At the Instituto di Medicina in Italy (*Metabolism* v 49, 2000) patients increased their glucose disposal and utilization simply by taking ALC, with no other changes in their diet or exercise. *Vegetarians, vegans, and macrobiotics should not take ALC, or any other animal protein, such as carnosine.* The research is very conflicting here.

Acidophilus is a probiotic supplement for all ages. Our digestive systems are generally in poor shape from our diet and lifestyle. Take one with six billion or more units and eight or more different strains. It must be bought and kept refrigerated like flax or fish oil. This is best used with FOS and l-glutamine for better digestion. If you feel your digestion is weak, take all three in both the AM and PM, for one year. Weekly fasting on water for one day every week is important here, to give your digestive system a rest 52 times a year. For even better results, join the Young Again international monthly two day fast. *Ninety percent of our immunity comes from our digestive system.* Better digestion equals stronger immunity. It works synergistically with aloe vera, too.

Beta-carotene is an important, basic antioxidant, and preferable to vitamin A. Beta-carotene is the precursor to vitamin A, and is safer and more effective. With blood sugar dysfunction you need all the known basic antioxidants. A time-proven vitamin, take 10,000 IU daily. Do not take any more than this. Antioxidants are central to curing oxidative stress and inflammation. Overdoses are always counterproductive; 10,000 IU is all you need.

Beta glucan *is the most effective immune enhancer known to science.* Our immunity is central to our health, and only a total program of diet and lifestyle will keep it strong. This is an important supplement for people of all ages. Just take 400 mg a day. You can take 800 mg a day for just one year if you like. All true glucans are equally effective, whether from oats, barley, mushrooms, or yeast. This has strong science behind it. Don't pay more than $10 for 60 X 400 mg. You can get grams of glucans by simply eating more oats and barley.

Beta-sitosterol is the most effective supplement known for lowering cholesterol and triglycerides. Take 300 mg a day. You can take 600 mg a day for a year if your cholesterol is over 200 mg/dl. The typical American diet only provides about 300 mg of mixed sterols. This is literally found in every vegetable you eat, but we eat few green and yellow vegetables. This is also the best single supplement to support good prostate and breast health, and is literally 1,000 times stronger than saw palmetto. There is great science behind plant sterols.

CoQ10 is very important for any cardiovascular issue. Take 100 mg and no less. This is not found in your food, and our levels fall as we age. Buy only real Japanese biosynthesized CoQ10. (Read the label to make sure.) Real CoQ10 is ubiquinone. *Do not buy ubiquinol,* as it is unstable with no shelf life. You can find 60 capsules for under $20. Take CoQ10 with food or flax oil, as it is oil soluble. Do not listen to any claims of "special delivery systems." There is excellent research on CoQ10 and hypertension, as well as on CHD health in general. There is no reason to take more, unless you have a serious heart condition. If you do, take 200 mg for one year. This is a most important supplement for anyone over 40.

DIM (di-indolyl methane) helps lower and normalize estrogen levels in men and women. This is a much better choice than indole3-carbinol. You must take 200 mg and no less. *"Special delivery systems"* are all scams. Just take this with your flax oil or food, as it is oil soluble. You can find 60 capsules of 200 mg for only about $12, if you Google "DIM." If your estradiol and estrone tests are in the low normal range (men or women) you do not need this. Low normal estradiol and estrone (and high normal estriol) are the ideal, based on rural Asian people, vegetarians, and macrobiotics. Sulforaphane is another effective natural aromatase inhibitor.

Flax oil is the best source of omega-3 fatty acids, and better than fish oil. *All studies on fish oil would apply equally to flax oil.* We have a serious imbalance of omega-6 to omega-3 fatty acids in our blood. Just read Chapter 11: Omega-3 Fatty Acids. The international clinical human evidence for the value of omega-3 fatty acids on blood pressure, insulin metabolism, and CHD health in general is overwhelming. Take a 1 gram capsule, or a half teaspoon of refrigerated "high lignan" liquid (1.5 grams). There is no reason to take more than this. Choose flax oil. *You must buy this and keep this refrigerated.* Never buy an unrefrigerated product.

FOS (fructooligosaccharides) is an indigestible prebiotic sugar that feeds the good bacteria in your digestive system. It is an extract of chicory root or the Terminalia plant. Take it with acidophilus and l-glutamine for good digestion. This is a supplement for all ages. Like glutamine, it is a prebiotic.

Glucosamine is a proven nutrient for bone and joint health. Do not spend your money on chondroitin, MSM, CLA, hyaluronic acid, and other unproven supplements. *Glucosamine does not work by itself.* You must use cofactors such as minerals, vitamins (especially vitamin D), flax oil, and hormones, such as progesterone, testosterone, and estriol (women). It takes time and patience to cure arthritis and other bone and joint conditions, as bone and cartilage grow slowly. Take 500 to 1,000 mg daily.

Glutamine is an amino acid that helps keep your digestive system healthy. You should take one gram a day as 500 mg tablets or capsules. Take it with acidophilus and FOS to insure good digestion. If you have a more serious digestive issue, buy bulk glutamine and take 3 grams a day for one year; then, 1 gram as maintenance. It has no real taste, and mixes easily with your food, or in soymilk. People under 40 can take this as well. AM and PM dosing is best.

Lipoic acid is a powerful supplement for blood sugar problems. Take 400 mg of regular lipoic acid. *The "R-only" form is expensive* and has no advantage at all. Nearly all the research is done on normal R,S-lipoic acid. This is not found in food, so you must supplement it. Insulin resistance is the basis of hypertension, and lipoic acid is vital here as part of a total program of maintaining low blood sugar and insulin levels. Lipoic acid works synergistically with minerals, flax oil, beta glucan, and other proven supplements.

Minerals. Please read Chapter 7: The Minerals You Need. You need at least 17 known FDA approved elements. Just search the Internet for "mineral supplements" to find one with 17 elements. People of all ages are mineral deficient, and need to supplement them. *Every medical condition known is due in part to mineral deficiency.* We all need a good mineral supplement.

NAC (N-acetyl cysteine) is the best way to raise your antioxidant glutathione level. Surprisingly, this works better than taking glutathione itself. Take 600 mg a day. More and more research keeps showing varied benefits for NAC supplementation, including increased immunity. We have animal studies on NAC and blood pressure, and soon we'll have human studies as well. Glutathione and SOD are your two major antioxidant enzymes.

Phosphatidyl serine (PS) is a relative of lecithin (phosphatidyl choline). It is a basic building block of brain cells. Take this along with pregnenolone and flax oil to insure good brain function, memory, clear thought, and cognition. The human studies for Alzheimer's are most impressive. Take 100 mg a day. This is now extracted from soybeans inexpensively, and it is an important supplement for everyone over 40 to maintain a strong, clear mind as you age.

Quercetin is a borderline antioxidant supplement, since it is mostly only found in apples and onions in any quantity. Definitely, take this for at least a year. The science is good, and it is a fine, but optional one to take in 100 mg doses. Most of the studies are on animals, but more and more good human ones are being done.

Soy isoflavones are a proven supplement with endless science behind them. Flavones are plant pigments, and not "phytoestrogens." (There are no hormones or pro-hormones in any plant.) Just take at least 40 mg of mixed genestein and daidzein. *If you use soy milk regularly you don't have to take this.* The popular anti-soy propaganda is all from the meat and dairy industries, especially the Weston Price Foundation. Billions of Asians over centuries prove that soy is good food. The Okinawans are the healthiest and longest-lived people on earth. They eat more soy foods than anyone. *Using soymilk is the most practical and realistic way to take them.*

Sulforaphane is a very powerful and effective supplement. A mere 1 mg (1,000 mcg) is all you need. The recent human published research is most impressive for a wide variety of health issues. It enhances immunity, and has anti-oxidant and anti-inflammatory properties. It is a natural aromatase inhibitor. It is a powerful supplement for preventing and curing blood sugar and insulin conditions. Like DIM, this is found naturally in cruciferous vegetables. You definitely want to take this.

Superoxide Dismutase (SOD) is the other basic antioxidant enzyme along with glutathione. Our blood and tissue SOD levels fall as we age. Low SOD is clearly correlated with hypertension and CHD conditions in general. It does not absorb, taken orally, and *all oral SOD supplements do not work.* Currently there is no practical way to take SOD, and doctors do not know how to inject it. Exercise, good diet, and natural hormone balance all help to keep your levels high.

VITAMINS

There are 13 known vitamins, so just take a good vitamin supplement. You must find one with 1 mg of methyl cobalamin, instead of regular B-12 (cyano cobalamin). Regular B-12 is simply not orally absorbable, so methyl cobalamin is the most effective way to do this. Do *not* take megadoses of any vitamins, as megadoses of anything just hurt your health. Do not take megadoses of any B-vitamin. People of all ages should take a good 13-vitamin supplement.

Vitamin C is totally optional. It can be taken as a 250 mg supplement, but no more than that. This is 400 percent of the RDA. This is completely optional. Megadoses of vitamin C will acidify your normally alkaline blood and make you sickly in the long run. *Do not take more than 250 mg of vitamin C!* The long-term side effects will do more harm than good. Antioxidants are a major part of lowering blood pressure, and vitamin C is one of our basic antioxidants. The only real source of vitamin C is tropical fruits.

Vitamin D can be taken as a 400 IU supplement, unless you are in the sun regularly. Vitamin D3 is really a hormone, not a vitamin. It must be emphasized that *vitamin D deficiency is a worldwide epidemic*. Taking a daily supplement can actually add years to your life. Vitamin D is not found in your food; you can only get it by exposure to the sun. *Do not take more than a total of 1,200 IU* (400 IU in your vitamin supplement and an extra 800 IU) if you are not in the sun. The 5,000 IU megadoses you see sold are toxic and dangerous.

Vitamin E can be taken as a 200 IU supplement; 200 IU is enough, and is seven times the RDA. Taking 400 IU long term thins your blood too much, and inhibits normal coagulation. You can simply take 400 IU every other day if you wish. Be sure to use the natural mixed tocopherols, and not the synthetic single d-alpha. The research on this is overwhelming, and goes back decades.

Scientists have only recently admitted this is vital for human nutrition.

CONCLUSION

Take the proven supplements outlined in this chapter for optimal health as part of a total program of diet and lifestyle. Natural supplements are a favorable way to maintain good health. The next chapter covers the endogenous supplements and the temporary supplements; temporary endogenous supplements and exogenous supplements

10. Temporary Supplements

Endogenous supplements are ones that exist naturally in our bodies and/or our daily food. These include all the ones mentioned in the previous chapter. Exogenous supplements are ones that do not exist naturally in our bodies or our daily food. This includes fruit pectin, ellagic acid, aloe vera, and curcumin. We are also going to discuss temporary endogenous supplements like taurine, TMG, and sodium alginate. All of these can be taken for six to twelve months only, and then discontinued. Exogenous supplements should be temporary.

ENDOGENOUS SUPPLEMENTS

Aloe vera is a time-proven remedy, especially for our digestion and liver functions. Take two capsules of 100 mg 200:1 extract. This equals 40 grams of fresh aloe gel. (Aloe gel is 99.5 percent water.) It works well with acidophilus, FOS, and l-glutamine.

Ellagic acid is found in black walnut hulls and other plants, such as Terminalia chebula. Make sure the label states that each capsule contains at least 100 mg of *actual* ellagic acid. Avoid overpriced raspberry seed products. It will not lower your blood pressure per se, but is a proven herbal supplement that will help your general health, and make you more resistant to cancer and other malignancies.

Fruit pectin from citrus or apples, taken as 3 grams a day (6 X 500 mg), is a very proven supplement for lowering blood fats. You can also use other plant polysaccharides, such as guar gum, glucomannon (konjac root), and sodium alginate (from seaweed). Avoid "modified" citrus pectin, which is an expensive and no better than plain pectin. The value of guar gum for lowering blood pressure, insulin, and blood sugar was proven at Royal Adelaide Hospital in 2003.

TEMPORARY ENDOGENOUS SUPPLEMENTS

Sodium alginate from seaweed is a proven way to reduce cholesterol and remove heavy metals like lead, cadmium, and mercury from your blood. Just take 3 grams (6 X 500 mg) for six months. Google this on the Internet, as it can be hard to find.

Taurine is endogenous, and is in your daily food. It has value for diabetes and hypertension. Both conditions often show low blood levels. It still should only be taken for a year in 1 to 2 gram doses. The science behind taurine and diabetes is strong. In 2004, an extensive review of the literature with 114 references at the University of Sassari was done. It demonstrated good benefits in treating diabetes and insulin resistance. You won't need this after you are well.

TMG (trimethylglycine) is the most powerful and effective liver rejuvenator known to science. Take 3 g (6 X 500 mg) for six to twelve months. You can take 1 g (2 X 500 mg) for the rest of your life if you want, which will help keep your homocysteine level low. Read the *Rejuvenate Your Liver* article found at our website.

EXOGENOUS SUPPLEMENT

Curcumin, 500 mg, is a well studied and time proven antioxidant from the tumeric root. It is exogenous, so some people will not be helped by taking it. You need all the antioxidants you can take when treating hypertension and insulin resistance, and this is a good one.

What about well advertised supplements that are supposed to work to lower blood pressure? Most of these are simply advertising promotions for profit, and not effective at all. Arginine is useless, no matter what you read somewhere. Theoretically, arginine is the precursor for nitrous oxide (NO). The only "studies" use insane over doses either orally or by infusion (drip injections) to get any effects. Thirty years of published research fails to show any value here for supplementation. Bitter Melon (Momordica) just has no science behind it.

Gymnema sylvestre is heavily promoted, but where are the studies? Lots of advertisements instead. Fenugreek seed also has advertisements instead of studies. Nopal cactus just has no proof of (2,600 mg) effectiveness. Cinnamon extract is also heavily promoted for blood sugar problems, but there are just no human studies to back this.

CONCLUSION

Temporary supplements are not even necessary, but can certainly speed your healing. Just remember they are temporary like for six months. Spend your time, effort, and money on the permanent ones.

11. Omega-3 Fatty Acids

Omega-3 fatty acids are so important they deserve a chapter of their own. Alpha linolenic acid (ALA) is very different from alpha linoleic acid (LA). ALA is found in plants, especially flax seed, walnuts, and black walnuts. EPA (eicosapentaneoic acid) and DHA (docohexanoic acid) are found abundantly in fish and seafood. Another name for omega-3 fatty acids is N-3 fatty acids. It does not matter whether we get our omega-3s from ALA or EPA/DHA. *We eat far too many omega-6 fatty acids, and far too few omega-3s.*

One reason is that we don't eat a natural foods diet. Another reason is Omega-3s are just not common in most foods in any quantity. If you eat walnuts every week you'll get plenty of ALA, but few people do that. If you eat seafood regularly you'll get plenty of EPA/DHA. Fatty fish, like salmon and tuna, have high omega-3s, but are 30 percent fat calories. You shouldn't be eating high-calorie, high-fat fish regularly anyway.

SOURCES FOR OMEGA-3 FATTY ACIDS

The most practical sources are fish oil and flax oil. Chia seed, krill, and hemp seed are also good sources, but impractical. You can also do this by eating 10 percent seafoods. The following are mg per 100 g portions: shrimp 400, salmon 1,100, tuna 1,300, whitefish 1,300, bluefish 1,200, oysters 500, pollack 500, rainbow trout 600, and cod 300 mg.

English walnuts contain an amazing 2.6 g (2,600 mg) of ALA per ounce! Black walnuts also very high in ALA.

Flax oil, is by far, the best choice, and is much preferable to fish oils. Flax has twice the omega-3 content of fish. Flax oil is less subject to oxidation by light, heat, and oxygen. Flax contains valuable lignans. Fish oil is more prone to oxidation. Flax oil is also much less expensive than fish oil, and it is easier to find refrigerated brands. Flax oil has a pleasant nutty taste, whereas fish oil must be taken in a softgel capsule. Fish oils also contain dangerous arachidonic acid. Blood levels of this are correlated with various diseases. Fish oil has no lignans. Flax is the best possible source of valuable plant lignans, which are an important, but deficient, part of our diet. We get very few vital lignans in our food. *Just choose refrigerated flax oil with lignans and keep it refrigerated. You can also buy a separate lignan supplement.*

Plant sources of supplements are always best when available, since a plant based diet is healthiest. Do not use expensive borage, black currant, or primrose oils, as they all have lower levels of omega-3s. Most of the studies on omega-3s use fish oil, *but all of these studies would equally apply to flax.* Any study that used fish oil would have gotten the same results with flax oil.

Whether you choose fish oil or flax oil, you must buy it and keep it refrigerated. Both have very short shelf lives, and *must be kept under refrigeration.* At room temperature they soon turn rancid, and then have lots of harmful free radicals.

Whether you are concerned about high cholesterol, triglycerides, C-reactive protein, homocysteine, heart attack, stroke, or any other heart and artery related problem, you must take flax oil. One to two grams should be enough. You can also use a half teaspoon (1.5 grams) of high-lignan liquid flax oil. There are only 9 calories in every gram of fish or flax oil, so this does not add to your caloric or fat intake. This is a supplement for people of all ages, including children. It is one of only eight supplements people under 40 need (along with vitamins, minerals, acidophilus, FOS, beta glucan, vitamin D, and vitamin E). You can also give this to your pets. The published human, clinical studies on omega-3 supplementation are overwhelming.

SCIENTIFIC RESEARCH ON OMEGA-3 FATTY ACIDS

A very good review from the University of Iowa (*Current Opinion in Lipidology* v 7, 1996), "N-3 Fatty Acids and Hypertension," was most convincing. It was substantiated by 37 references. They clearly stated, "N-3 fatty acid supplementation reduced blood pressure in patients with essential hypertension." Some of the studies reviewed found omega-3 supplementation made hypertension drugs more effective. This is not recommended at all, since you should do this naturally *without any drugs.* Other studies found heart transplant patients on anti-rejection drugs fared better by taking omega-3s. They also found omega-3s caused vasorelaxation to expand the blood vessels and allow better blood flow.

A very long 14 page review, with 96 references, was published in *Annals of the NY Academy of Sciences* (v 827, 1997). This is a highly sophisticated article written in very technical language, and meant for professionals. The bottom line, however, is that *omega-3 supplementation lowers blood pressure,* and is good for overall heart and artery health. They point out that both fish and flax oils are the best sources of omega-3s, with flax oil containing the most, at about 50 percent. They also showed omega-3s help prevent the development of proteinuria (high protein in the blood, especially albumin, from kidney dysfunction). "Reduction of dietary fat, particularly saturated fat, is a key strategy for preventing cardiovascular disease, but it is unlikely to lower blood pressure unless accompanied by weight loss." They emphasized the need for high blood omega-3 levels to keep blood pressure down.

At the University of Tromso (*Annals of Internal Medicine* v 123, 1995) men and women were given expensive DHA/EPA capsules in a classic double blind, placebo study. It would have been more practical to give them inexpensive flax oil. Both diastolic and systolic pressures were lowered significantly, with no change in diet, lifestyle, or exercise. Both triglycerides and low-density (LDL) cholesterol levels also fell significantly. At the University of Trondheim (*16th Scandinavian Symposium on Lipids,* 1991) people were given omega-3 fatty acid supplements. Their blood pressure fell significantly with no other treatments.

At the University of Florence (*Thrombosis Research* v 91, 1998) they stated clearly, "Dietary n-3 polyunsaturated fatty acids can lower blood pressure in humans." Here healthy controls were compared to hypertensives, with very good results in only 60 days. At Yokosuka Research Group in Japan (*Journal of Oleo Science* v 56, 2007) they said, "These results suggest that ALA (alpha linolenic acid) has an antihypertensive effect with no adverse effect in subjects with high-normal blood pressure and mild hypertension." At Shimane Medical University in Japan they found, "Increased dietary n-3 PUFA intakes from marine fish and plants may modify the blood pressure and risk factors for CVD and decrease the incidence of CVD."

At Lok Nayak Hospital in India (*Indian Journal of Clinical Biochemistry* v 20, 2005) 100 patients were given real flax oil supplements for only 4 weeks. "A significant reduction of fasting plasma insulin levels in both groups was observed (29.0 percent and 22.8 percent) as well as serum cholesterol, triglyceride, and LDL, while HDL rose 8 percent in both groups." This kind of dramatic effect with flax oil alone is nothing less than amazing. They recommended routine flax supplementation, and curtailment of omega-6 intake for hypertension.

At the Barzilai Medical Center in Israel, omega-3s were given to hypertensives. "Dietary supplementation with n-3 PUFA decreases blood pressure and serum triglycerides. In both non-diabetics and diabetics, similar significant decreases in blood pressure were achieved with no other intervention."

At the University of Trondheim they said, "The results

therefore indicate that long-chain n-3 fatty acids probably have the same (positive) effect on blood pressure irrespectively of whether they are taken as fish oil or part of the normal Norwegian diet."

A thorough review (*Omega-3 Fatty Acids,* Drevon 1993), with 18 references, went into great detail on the mechanisms for the blood pressure lowering effect of omega-3 fatty acids. The University of Colorado (*Journal of Hypertension* 19, 2001) said omega-3 supplements reduced insulin resistance. At Weizmann Institute in Israel (*Journal of Clinical and Basic Cardiology* v 5, 2002) people given an omega-3 supplement, and a diet low in omega-6s, benefited greatly. "In the n-3 group we observed a significant decrease of serum cholesterol, LDL, triglyerides, and insulin. Hypertension, which was positively correlated to hyper-insulemia, decreased significantly, especially the systolic."

The Institute of Military Hygeine in China (*Yingyang Xuebao* v 14, 1992) gave EPA and DHA to hypertensives for only 10 weeks. "In vitro thrombosis was remarkably inhibited in subjects, and systolic and diastolic blood pressure were markedly lowered." No other treatment but omega-3 supplementation.

The most important study of all (*British Journal of Diabetes* v 8, 2008) showed simply that *blood levels of omega-3 fatty acids were clearly correlated with all cause mortality!* The higher the level of omega-3s in your body, the longer you'll live and the healthier you'll be. This shows just how important omega-3 supplements are. This is a supplement for all ages—and your pets.

CONCLUSION

Omega-3 fatty acid supplements are vital, not only to a program of treating hypertension, but treating all forms of coronary heart conditions. *Omega-3s are heart and artery healthy!* Coronary heart disease is the biggest killer of all by far.

In the next chapter you will learn about the importance of exercise, aerobic or cardiovascular, in lowering your blood pressure and making your heart stronger.

12. You Must Exercise

Y ou can literally cure cancer while sitting on the couch watching television all day. Of course, it is always better to exercise, and your healing will go much better and much faster if you do exercise. Really vigorous exercise is best, but just walking a half hour a day is all you really need. *Exercise is absolutely vital.*

With hypertension, insulin resistance, and diabetes you *must* exercise to get well. There is no way around this. Lack of exercise is a major cause of high blood pressure. In rural agrarian societies, one reason hypertension is so rare is due to the great amount of physical work required just to survive and eat. Exercise is so powerful and so effective that some people can cure their hypertension with just vigorous exercise, such as walking, jogging, jumping rope, bicycling, skating, rowing, low-impact or high-impact aerobics, and swimming, with no other change in diet or lifestyle. That is not the sermon in this book at all. This is said simply to stress how vital regular daily exercise is to maintaining normal blood pressure levels.

The published clinical studies are overwhelming. Exercise lowers both systolic and diastolic pressures very dramatically, but does much more than that. It improves many biological diagnostic parameters as well, as we'll see in the following studies.

SCIENTIFIC RESEARCH
TO PROVE THE IMPORTANCE OF EXERCISE

At the University of Tennessee (*Preventive Medicine* v 37, 2003) doctors simply had the patients walk every day, with no other changes in their lifestyles. For eight weeks they simply walked a lot every day. Their blood pressure fell dramatically.

At Kyushi University in Japan (*Metabolism, Clinical & Experimental* v. 51, 2002) diabetic hypertensive men used an exercise bike every day. It was harder to lower blood pressure in diabetics because of their generally poor physical condition. They were given glucose tolerance tests (GTT) that showed improved insulin resistance. They also lowered both systolic and diastolic pressures with no other lifestyle changes.

Beta endorphins are the "feel good hormone" that fill our opioid receptors. Exercise raises beta endorphin levels, and makes us feel good naturally. Male hypertensives at the Second Military Medical University in China (*Shanghai Yixue* v 17, 1994) were found to be low in beta endorphins. Two weeks of mild exercise raised their beta endorphin levels, lowered their blood pressure, and the men had a greater feeling of well being with no other lifestyle changes.

At St. Thomas Hospital in London (*Circulation* v 101, 2000) male hypertensives were found to have insulin resistance as well as high total cholesterol levels. "Changes in diastolic blood pressure during gentle exercise are strongly associated with serum concentrations of total cholesterol and insulin resistance. This may contribute to development of hypertensive complications in dyslipidemic and/or insulin resistant patients." Notice this was merely "gentle exercise," and not rigorous at all.

Russian doctors (*Eksperimental'naya Meditsina* v 26, 1991) found hypertensives had decreased exercise tolerance and high blood lactate levels. Regular exercise gave them a greater ability to exercise longer and dispose of excess lactic acid. Exercise reduces hyper levels of lactic acid in the blood. This builds up as hypertension reduces the body's ability to dispose of it.

A really thorough review, "Antihypertensive Mechanism of Exercise," was done at Fukuoka University in Japan (*Journal of Hypertension* v 11, 1993) complete with 69 references. The urban Japanese (not the rural) have the highest blood pressure in the world. Here, studies around the world were collected. The doctors were primarily interested in understanding exactly how exercise lowers blood pressure, and which mechanisms were responsible. They studied such exotic parameters as noepinephrine, kallikrein, prostaglandin E, natriuretic peptide, dopamine, and ouabain. This gets pretty technical, but the bottom line is that exercise works well, and we don't need to worry about the hows and whys. After reading such a thorough and well documented review, there is no doubt left as to how effective and necessary any kind of exercise is.

At Katedra i Klinika Kardiology in Poland (*Polskie Archiwum Medycyny Wewnetrznej* v 104, 2000) men and women with hypertension were found to have hyper leptin levels. They found, "The moderate, short-term exercise decreases serum leptin levels in the hypertensive patients." Here, exercise was found not only to lower blood pressure, but leptin levels as well.

At the Medical University of Warsaw (*Journal of Human Hypertension* v 12, 1998) hypertensive men were given a daily exercise program. *One single bout of exercise lowered their blood pressure significantly.* This phenomenon has been found in other studies as well. They did a 20-minute session daily on an exercise-bicycle (ergometer). The doctors concluded, "Long lasting antihypertensive effect of a single dynamic exercise in hypertensives suggests that moderate exercise may be applied as an effective physiological procedure to reduce elevated arterial blood pressure in mild hypertension." Notice the term "long lasting."

At Computense University (*Antioxidants* 7, 2005) they strongly link oxidative stress and inflammation to hypertension. Exercise is very powerful for reducing both oxidative stress and inflammation. They show that exercise is a vital part of any blood pressure lowering program.

At Ohio University (*Comparative Biochemistry* v 133C, 2002) the doctors also found that exercise improved antioxidant levels and reduced oxidative stress. This led to lower blood pressure with no other changes in diet or lifestyle.

At Taipei Medical University (*Clinical and Experimental Hypertension* v 24, 2002) they found: "Moderate intensity regular exercise training in these patients reduces blood pressure." Here, just 12 weeks of using a treadmill reduced systolic pressure a whopping 18 mm with no change in diet. *An 18 mm drop is simply amazing.* Total cholesterol, LDL, and triglycerides were reduced, and HDL raised significantly.

At the University of Naples (*Journal of Human Hypertension* v 17, 2003) more work was done in this area. "The results demonstrate that exercise is associated with enhanced blood nitrosation, and suggest that the ascorbate, or urate, levels increase to limit oxidative damage." In plain words, exercise greatly improved antioxidant function, and oxidative stress was reduced remarkably. They measured six different antioxidant levels in their blood, and found all of them to rise after a mild exercise program. Exercise raises antioxidants!

We discussed that insulin sensitivity is at the heart of rising blood pressure. Exercise improves insulin sensitivity greatly. At the University of Michigan (*Metabolism, Clinical and Experimental* v 53, 2004) this was proven with elderly men and women. Older people are much harder to treat. "In conclusion, a 4-month resistance training program significantly increased insulin-mediated glucose disposal and lean body mass . . . in older hypertensive subjects."

At the Laval University (*Circulation* v 108, 2003) doctors noted that two causes of hypertension are reduced glycogen (stored source of blood sugar) synthesis and insulin sensitivity. Mild exercise of any kind raises both very effectively.

At the University of Tsukuba (*Hypertension Research* v. 27, 2004) two separate studies were published. In the first, postmenopausal women did low intensity aerobic cycle-exercise for

12 weeks. Their blood pressure fell significantly. In the second, more elderly women did moderate cycle exercise. Their nitric oxide (NOx) blood levels rose while their blood pressure fell. NOx is very important to keeping blood pressure low, and falls as we age. In the same journal a year later (v. 28) they verified the positive effect of exercise on NOx. They also found their superoxide dismutase (SOD) levels rose as well. *Exercise raises SOD!* "Lifestyle modification is recommended as a non-pharmacological approach to treatment of hypertension," they said. The urban Japanese have the highest blood pressure in the world despite their generally good diet. More and more they adopt the Western ways of high-sugar and high-fat refined foods and suffer the consequences. The rural Japanese tend to remain healthy.

At Kansai Medical University (*Clinical and Experimental Hypertension* v 19, 1997) people with hypertension exercised for three months. Of course their blood pressure fell, but other sophisticated blood parameters were very much improved as well.

CONCLUSION

Exercise is simply good for your entire health. When you exercise, everything in your body improves in both overt and subtle ways. *You must exercise to lower your blood pressure.* There is no way around this. You can do aerobic or resistance, and you can do low or high intensity. Join a gym if you can, or put equipment in your home. Or you can just take a brisk walk every day. Thomas Jefferson said, "The sovereign invigorator of the body is exercise and, of all the exercises, walking is the best." Do what you enjoy best. Yes, you will come to enjoy your daily workouts.

13. Your Basic Hormones

Maintaining a youthful hormone level is a basic part of real macrobiotics, natural health, longevity, and life extension. Doctors, including endocrinologists, have very little knowledge of natural hormone balance. This includes naturopaths, holistic, and life extension specialists. You have to depend on yourself and use saliva testing and online blood labs. Medical doctors are just not trained in natural hormone balance, your basic hormones, how to measure them, or how to balance them.

BASIC HORMONES

Hormones, like minerals, work together as a team harmoniously and synergistically in concert. We want to have all of our 14 basic hormones at youthful levels as much as possible. We need to go far beyond merely balancing insulin and blood sugar, as all our hormones work together and support each other. Let's look at the basic fourteen:

1. Androstenedione
2. Cortisol
3. DHEA
4. Estradiol
5. Estriol
6. Estrone

7. Growth Hormone

8. Insulin

9. Melatonin

10. Pregnenolone

11. Progesterone

12. T3

13. T4

14. Testosterone

Androstenedione

Androstenedione (and androstenediol) is the direct precursor to testosterone. The blood level generally parallels that of testosterone. Men don't need to measure this, and women only need to measure this if they have high testosterone and/or DHEA, which indicates androgenicity. Using androstenedione, androstenediol, or their analogs is not a good way to raise testosterone, and they are now classified as prescription drugs.

Cholesterol

Cholesterol is, in fact, the "grandmother" of hormones from which all the sex hormones are made. This is the starting point. Along with your triglycerides, cholesterol is the best indicator of coronary heart health. CRP (C-reactive protein), uric acid, and homocysteine are the other three.

It is important to maintain low levels using diet, supplements, hormones, exercise, and regular short term fasting. *Your total cholesterol level should be about 150 mg/dl.* Yes, this is a realistic goal, and billions of rural Asians prove that it is. Your triglycerides should be under 100. The *only* way to raise cholesterol is by eating the saturated animal fat found in red meat, poultry, eggs, and dairy products. Triglycerides are raised by eating too much of any simple sugars, including honey or fruit juice.

Cortisol

Cortisol is the stress hormone. Very little research has been done on naturally normalizing cortisol levels. *You really don't even need to test your cortisol levels.* Basically cortisol is what it is. Only diet and lifestyle is going to normalize your cortisol levels.

We need more research on practical application, since our levels vary widely during a 24-hour period. This is why only a four-sample saliva test can give you an accurate profile of this variance. You can do a 12-hour profile at 9/1/5/9, but this just isn't necessary. Yes, cortisol levels are correlated with high blood pressure.

At the 401 Hospital in China (*Zhongguo Kangfu* v 8, 2004), hypertensive men showed high cortisol readings along with depression and anxiety.

At the University of New South Wales (*Steroids* v 60, 1995), an extensive review was done with 34 references showing hypertension is highly correlated with high cortisol levels. They said this is characterized by sodium retention.

At Hubei Central Hospital (*Fangshe Zazhi* v 20, 2007), patients were tested at 8 AM, 4 PM, and midnight for a daily profile. "Marked elevated plasma cortisol levels were observed in patients with essential hypertension and coronary heart disease."

DHEA

DHEA is the other major androgen. It is known as the "life extension hormone," for good reason. Youthful levels are strongly correlated with good health and long life. There are countless published international human studies showing how vital this is. Dramatic results are found with proper supplementation.

In men and women this is often deficient after the age of 40. In women of any age DHEA can also be excessive, as well as deficient. This condition is called androgenicity, and high testosterone and androstenedione are often found as well. Look for the level you had at about age 30. To know your level you never, never take DHEA without prior blood or saliva testing. Men who prove low can take 25 mg, and women who are low can take 12.5 mg (half-tablets). DHEA, like pregnenolone, is only about 10 percent absorbed when taken orally. The only way to lower excessive levels is by diet, exercise, and lifestyle, as well as balancing your other hormones.

Estradiol

Estradiol (E2) is the strongest and most dangerous of the three basic estrogens. Men over 50 literally have higher levels of estradiol than their postmenopausal wives!

Western women generally have excessive E2 levels due to high fat consumption, obesity, and lack of exercise. These are major causes of breast, cervical, and ovarian cancers. One-third of U.S. women will willingly be castrated, which destroys their total hormone balance. *All hysterectomies atrophy the ovaries*, which means diminished hormone production. You want low-normal levels and not midrange ones. You almost never find a woman low in estradiol even after a hysterectomy.

At Laiwu People's Hospital (*Fangshe Zazhi* v 19, 2006) both male and female hypertensives were shown to have high estradiol levels. "The authors suggested that the changes of serum sex hormones levels might be a risk factor rather than a consequence of essential hypertension."

At the General Hospital in Beijing (*Zhonghua Zazhi* v 9, 2007) men were found to have high estradiol and high estrogen-to-testosterone ratios. Young men have a healthy reversed ratio where testosterone dominates estradiol and estrone. In men testosterone should always dominate.

Estriol

Estriol, like pregnenolone, is the forgotten or orphan hormone, even though it comprises 80 percent of human estrogen. This only applies to women. Doctors almost never test women for it, never prescribe it, and the word "estriol" is really not even in their vocabulary. Studies have shown up to 100 percent of obese women are deficient in estriol. Doctors know very little about estriol.

Amazingly enough, you cannot buy, or even special order, estriol in regular pharmacies! This shows that the pharmaceutical world is in the Dark Ages. Only the compounding pharmacies can make this up, but they extort you by selling 50 cents worth for $50.

You can find this on the Internet with 150 mg (0.25 percent) in 2 ounce creams for $20. The label must say 150 mg in 2 oz. This is the "safe" or "good" estrogen. Asian and vegetarian women have higher levels. You want high normal levels and not merely midrange ones. You only need to add about 500 mcg (0.5 mg) a day in your blood, if you test low by blood or saliva diagnosis.

Estrone

Estrone (E1) is the second strongest and, potentially, most dangerous of the three basic estrogens. Like estradiol, men over 50 literally have higher levels of estrone than their postmenopausal wives!

Supposedly, women in America and Europe are estrogen-deficient as they age, and need supplementation of estradiol and estrone. The truth is that Western women generally have excessive E1 levels, due to high fat consumption, obesity, and lack of exercise. This is also a major cause of various female cancers, such as uterine, breast, cervical, and ovarian. Since one-third of American women get hysterectomies, many of these women have low estriol and progesterone levels. Again, you want *low normal levels,* and not just midrange ones. What is considered "normal" in Western medicine is actually excessive. Rural Asian and African women have lower estradiol and estrone levels, and higher estriol and progesterone levels. Rural Asian men also have lower estradiol and estrone levels than Western men. It is rare to find a woman with low estrone levels. Transdermal estrone is not sold in pharmacies.

Growth Hormone

Growth hormone (GH) is very overrated, mostly because it is expensive and some movie stars use it. It is expensive because it is very difficult to biosynthesize this 192-amino acid chain molecule. Those over 50 can get moderate benefits from using GH. Our levels fall from the time we're teenagers until we're 80 or older, when GH almost disappears.

You get mild benefits here even when paying at least $120 a month to inject 1 IU daily. Yes, you must inject 1 IU subcutaneously (under your skin) every day. It only lasts one week refrigerated after diluting it, and the molecule breaks if you stir or shake it. Do not expect anything dramatic here, just because you are spending a lot of money. *Do not even think of taking this until every one of your basic hormones is balanced.* Don't even consider it. It is very difficult to get today unless you pay a doctor and a pharmacist hundreds of dollars a month for testing, prescriptions, and actual GH. You can order it online legally from offshore pharmacies for personal use. No over the counter GH precursor has any value at all.

Insulin

Insulin levels are very easy and inexpensive to measure with a fasting serum blood test. With hypertension, the most important hormone we need to deal with is insulin. Knowing your insulin level is vital. *You want a fasting serum level of about 5.0 µU/ml.* Most Americans have a level of about 9. The average Japanese person has a level of about 4.8. The standard medical reference range is far too high. This may sound difficult, but you can do this with diet and lifestyle; 5.0 µU/ml or less.

Know your blood sugar level. *Your fasting blood sugar should be 85 or less.* Please remember that figure—85 or less. Do not let the doctor tell you that higher values of, "100 or less" are all right. You can do this with an inexpensive non-coded meter.

If fasting sugar is over 85 mg/dl, then a glucose tolerance test (GTT) is called for. This is the gold standard, and tells you how effectively your insulin is reacting to the cells in your body. The GTT reveals insulin resistance better than any other test. It should be routine for anyone over 40. The GTT is accurate, inexpensive, non-invasive, and very underutilized. A two-hour glucose tolerance test (GTT) is the best test of all here. This tells you insulin response, and not just insulin levels. Your fasting blood sugar is tested. You drink a 75 g cup of glucose solution, wait two hours, and have your blood sugar tested again. You want a level 10 points below the accepted Western level—*at least 10 points under the accepted norm.* Some people have normal blood sugar levels, but are still insulin resistant. The GTT is accurate, inexpensive, and very worth doing.

The HbA1c is also a fine test to verify this. You can buy inexpensive test kits in your drug store. This shows your six month average of hemoglobin "glycation" (bonding to glucose). *Your HbA1c level should be 4.6 percent or less.* Yes, that is the correct number, not the normally accepted medical level of under 5.6 percent. Please remember that figure—4.6 percent.

Melatonin

Melatonin is a powerful antioxidant hormone. People don't understand how important and powerful it really is. This is a very underrated hormone, and science discovers new benefits for it every month.

Our levels fall from the time we reach twenty, and almost disappear by the time we're seventy. Most everyone over the age of 40 can, and should, take this. Take melatonin at night only and never during the day. The science about melatonin grows all the time, and now it is being used to both to prevent and to treat cancers of various kinds. Fortunately, we now have both animal and human studies to demonstrate just how important melatonin is in maintaining healthy blood pressure levels. It is not well known at all that melatonin is important for hypertension.

At the Netherlands Institute for Brain Research (*Hypertension* v 43, 2004), male hypertensives were given 2.5 mg melatonin every night for only three weeks. This was a classic double-blind, placebo-controlled study. "Repeated melatonin intake reduced systolic and diastolic blood pressure . . . and also improved sleep."

At Policlinico di Modena (*American Journal of Hypertension* v. 18, 2005), women were given melatonin for just three weeks in a randomized, crossover, double-blind study. "These data indicate that prolonged administration of melatonin may improve the day-night rhythm of blood pressure, particularly in women with a blunted nocturnal decline."

At the Cincinnati College of Medicine (*Journal of Pineal Research* v 36, 2004), type 1 diabetic hypertensive adolescents (average age only sixteen) were given melatonin for a week. These poor children had high blood pressure in addition to type 1 diabetes. Their blood pressure improved in only a week. The fact you can successfully treat children with melatonin is nothing less than amazing.

At the Zabreze Biochemical Clinic, men and women hypertensives, with an average age of forty-two, were given melatonin. One-third were severe, one-third were moderate, and one-third were healthy. "Results of our studies seem to confirm the concept that decreased melatonin secretion can be one of the causes of hypertension."

Pregnenolone

Pregnenolone is the forgotten, or "orphan," hormone, because so little work has been done studying it in clinics around the world. It is known as the "mother hormone," since the rest of the sex hormones are derived from it. This is *the* most important brain, memory, and cognition hormone, yet there is little research being done even today. It is best used with PS (phosphatidyl serine) and flax oil. There are no studies on the relation of pregnenolone levels to blood pressure, for the simple reason there is hardly any research at all on pregnenolone. In the future we will have such research. Youthful levels are necessary for total hormone balance.

Pregnenolone falls in men and women at about age forty, then levels off, and stays low the rest of one's life. Currently no saliva home tests are offered on the Internet. You can get an inexpensive blood test from an online lab without a doctor like www.healthlabs.com. Generally, men over forty can safely take 50 milligrams, and women 25 milligrams. As with DHEA, men have much higher levels of this. Only about 10 percent of pregnenolone (and DHEA) is absorbed when taken orally. This is the only practical way to take them however. Since all your hormones work together harmoniously in concert as a team in harmony, a youthful level of pregnenolone is absolutely vital.

Progesterone

Progesterone is important for both men and women. It is what balances the powerful estrogens, estradiol and estrone. Many premenopausal women are low in progesterone and don't know it. The ovaries stop producing it after menopause. Natural progesterone cream with 1,000 mg per two-ounce jar is readily available over the counter. Premenopausal women can use this two weeks of every cycle; postmenopausal women can choose any two weeks of the calendar month to use it; and men can use it five days a week. Progesterone is very safe, and there is no need to measure your level. Saliva testing is not effective here, as it is fat-soluble and requires a blood serum (not plasma) test.

T3 (triiodothyronine) and T4 (L-thyroxine)

T3 (triiodothyronine) and *T4* (L-thyroxine) are your basic thyroid hormones. You will get more dramatic effects from raising low thyroid levels than with any other hormone. This is where doctors and endocrinologists are really uninformed.

Measure your free T3 and free T4. Your TSH is what it is, and can only be lowered or raised with diet and lifestyle. Your free T3 and T4 tell you what you need to know. You want average, midrange values, and not merely "in range" values (add high and low range, and divide by two). Low normal values are known as "subclinical hypothyroidism." Doctors rarely measure free T3 and free T4, and they tell you that any in range value is acceptable. If you are low in either, or both, of these you will get more dramatic results for your money than with any other hormone.

You must treat T3 and T4 separately. Do not take Armour® or other animal extracts. Use generic versions of Synthroid® and Cytomel®, such as Levoxyl and Tiromel. These are both bioidentical in every way. There is a classic 4:1 ratio in mammals of L-throxine to triiodothyronine.

At Lanzhou Medical College the doctors said, "Thyroid hormone levels are closely correlated with age, and age is an independent influencing thyroid hormone factor in patients with essential hypertension." They found T3 and T4 to be very influential here. The same situation was discovered at Harvard University. "The authors have found that free T4 is lower and TSH is higher in hypertensives compared with normotensive euthyroid (healthy) subjects." Low thyroid has been associated with aortic stiffness, an important factor in hypertension. Anyone over 40 should know their thyroid hormone levels and balance them.

Testosterone

Testosterone is the basic androgen, along with DHEA and androstenedione. Women have only one tenth the amount, but it is just as vital to their health. Men cannot have hyper levels, as they cannot overproduce it. Even if they over supplement it, this just spills over into estrogens. Hyper levels in women can only be lowered by diet, exercise, and lifestyle, along with balancing the other hormones. Testosterone is very influential in diabetes and insulin resistance. *Hypertensive men are often deficient, while women are often excessive.* Men and women are very different here. Ninety-five per cent of normal, healthy men over 50 need supplementation anyway. That's right, 19 out of 20 men over the age of 50 are testosterone deficient, and they should raise their levels. Many women are deficient past menopause.

There are a wealth of studies showing male hypertensives are low in testosterone. Men who prove to be low can supplement with 3 mg of testosterone (4 mg of transdermal enanthate) in their blood.

There is little research on women here. It seems high

testosterone is often the issue with them. Women who prove to be low can supplement with 150 mcg of testosterone (200 mcg of transdermal enanthate) in their blood. Women who have an excessive level can only lower it with a program of diet and lifestyle. There are no safe drugs to lower testosterone. Any man or woman over 40 should test their *free* testosterone level (not bound or total), and make sure it is at a youthful level. The most famous study was done at the University of Tromso with 1,548 men (*European Journal of Endocrinology* v 150, 2004). "The results of the present study are consistent with the hypothesis that lower levels of testosterone in men are associated with higher blood pressure."

CONCLUSION

Taking toxic, dangerous drugs to lower your blood pressure merely covers up the symptoms and ignores the cause. Treat the cause of your problem with diet and lifestyle. Natural hormone balance is a vital part of this. All medical conditions are due in part to hormone imbalance. Your hormones work together synergistically as a team.

Hypertension really is a "silent killer." It is crucial to have your blood pressure under control, and this includes testing your hormone levels. The following chapter introduces you to a number of ways to test your basic hormone levels at home.

14. Home Hormone Testing

You do not need to see a doctor to test your hormones. It is very expensive to see one, and they usually are very poorly educated about natural hormone balance. This includes gynecologists, endocrinologists, naturopaths, holistic physicians, and life extension specialists.

TESTING OUR BASIC HORMONES

Let's go over how to test your basic hormones.

Androstenedione

Androstenedione does not have to be tested by men. Women can test this if they are high or low in either testosterone or DHEA. There is no need to take an androstenedione supplement, even if low, as your testosterone supplement will raise this naturally. Look for the youthful level you had at age 30.

DHEA

DHEA can be tested with saliva as free DHEA. Look for the youthful level you had at age 30. If low, men can take 25 mg orally, and women half-tablets of 12.5 mg. (Women only have about half men's blood level). It is only about 10 percent absorbed, so men get about 2.5 mg in their blood, and women about 1.25 mg. Men should test about 6 or higher on the ZRT scale, and women about 3. The high teenage levels cannot be regained after the age of 40 as with the other hormones, due to metabolic changes as we age.

Cholesterol

Cholesterol can be tested at home fairly accurately with test kits. You can use an online lab, rather than a regular lab, for $30. If you do this be sure to add a list of other tests mentioned in this book, such as triglyerides, CRP, uric acid, and homocysteine. Your level must be about 150 mg/ dl, and your triglycerides under 100.

Cortisol

Cortisol, like GH, needs a four draw comprehensive profile, but with a saliva kit at 9/1/5/9. *You just do not need to do this.* The only way to normalize your cortisol it is with diet, exercise, lifestyle, and balancing your other hormones. Cortisol varies greatly in most people during different times of the day. There is little research, and no real means for balancing cortisol.

Estradiol

Estradiol (E2) is almost never needed in any woman, even after a hysterectomy. Use a saliva test kit. *You want low normal values,* not normal or higher; 0.5 on the ZRT scale for men and post-meno-pausal women is the ideal. Men should test this, as high E2 is common in those over 50. If a woman is low, use a mere 10 mcg (micrograms) in your blood transdermally with DMSO, or sublingually in vegetable oil. Transdermal patches are very overpriced and very powerful. *Never use oral estradiol of any type.*

Estriol

Estriol is very often low in American and European women. Use a saliva test kit. *You want high normal values.* Men do not need to test this. If the test says you are under a certain point, but does not state the actual level, then assume you are low.

If low, use 500 mcg (0.5 mg) in DMSO or sublingually. Or use a 0.25 percent cream (150 mg in 2 ounces). Patches are not available, and never take oral estriol salts. Estriol is the predominant, and "safe" or "good" estrogen, but little research has been done.

This is the most abundant estrogen in both men and women. *Never use oral estriol of any type.* Low estriol is epidemic in women, especially in those who are overweight (1/3 of American women). The ZRT range of "under 7" is meaningless.

Estrone

Estrone (E1) is rarely needed in women, even after a hysterectomy. Use a saliva test kit. *You want low normal values;* 1.3 on the ZRT scale for men and postmenopausal women. Men should test this, as high E1 is common in men over 50. If a woman is low, use a mere 100 mcg (micrograms) in DMSO transdermally or sublingually in vegetable oil. Transdermal patches are very overpriced. *Never use oral estrone of any type.* E1 and E2 are prescription drugs.

GH

GH (*Growth Hormone*) cannot be tested by saliva, and it may be years before saliva kits are available. Ironically, accurate IGF-1 kits are available. *IGF-1 does not parallel GH,* and anyone who says it does is totally misinformed. You would need to go to a clinic for a 9/1/5/9 four-draw comprehensive profile. None of this is necessary. Are you over 50, and can afford $1,800 a year or more? Go by real-world results if you do. This is the most overrated hormone of all, simply because it is expensive. You can use 1 IU of GH daily sublingually dissolved in DMSO, but this is not legal and you would have to make it yourself. Shaking or stirring GH will break the molecule and make it useless. Balance all your other basic hormones before even considering this. It is only expensive since making long 192 amino acid chains is so difficult.

Insulin

Insulin uses a fasting serum blood test. Use an online lab like www.healthlabs.com without a doctor for $30. You want a result of 5.0 or less. You also want to test your blood sugar. Fasting glucose should be 85 or less.

Buy a non-coded meter at the drug store for $20. You will need a doctor for an accurate, non-invasive, inexpensive GTT (Glucose Tolerance Test). You want a result at least 10 points lower than the medically accepted ideal. Always remember that glucose/insulin metabolism is central to maintaining normal blood pressure levels. Insulin resistance and blood sugar dysmetabolism are the basic keys to understanding hypertension. Ask your doctor for a GTT the next time you have an annual checkup. Also check your HbA1c. Buy a $30 HbA1c kit at the drug store and get a six month average of your blood sugar glycation (bonding).

Melatonin

Melatonin has to be tested at home at 3:00 AM. There are very few saliva kits offered on the Internet. If you are over 40, men can safely take 3 mg at night only, and women can take half tablets of 1.5 mg, as their levels are lower.

The media have damned melatonin with faint praise as a mere sleep aid and for jet lag. The clinical facts are that this is a powerful antioxidant that helps regulate and slow down our biological aging clock. Melatonin has powerful anti-cancer and other dramatic properties. The more we study this, the more impressive the evidence is. Test with saliva at 3:00 in the morning. People over 40 should be able to use it without testing.

Pregnenolone

Pregnenolone levels can only be tested with a blood test. You can use an online lab for $50 with no doctor. Men over 40 can generally take 50 mg and women 25 mg. Only about 10 percent will actually be absorbed into your blood. The only practical way to take pregnenolone (or DHEA) is orally. You can't use either transdermally (across the skin) or sublingually (under the tongue) as they will not dissolve in vegetable oil, DMSO, or alcohol. In the future we'll have home saliva testing.

Progesterone

Progesterone does not need to be tested in women over 40, or in men. They just need to use it properly. Any woman who's had a hysterectomy should use this. *Saliva is not the way to test progesterone*, since it is oil soluble and can only be measured by (fatty) blood serum, not (watery) blood plasma.

Men can use a mere 1/8th teaspoon five days a week on the skin like their inner wrists. Premenopausal women will use this properly with their cycle. Remember that most all women over 40 have stopped ovulating, and no longer produce any significant amount of progesterone. Many younger women can also benefit from using this.

T3 And T4

T3 and T4 cannot currently be tested by saliva. You can use home blood spot tests for $85. You can use an online lab without a doctor though for the same price. In the future we should again have reliable, inexpensive saliva kits to test for free T3 and T4.

You must test your free T3 and free T4 (and TSH if you wish to add that). You can also see a doctor, but clearly demand free T3 and free T4, not TSH and T3 uptake. Again, do not accept "in range values." Just add high and low range and divide by two. *You must be midrange, and not merely in range.* There are no universal ranges here, and most labs differ. You can legally buy thyroid hormones online for personal use from offshore pharmacies. Look for T3 as Tiromel and T4 as Levoxyl and other generics.

Testosterone

Testosterone must be tested for your free, not bound or total form. *You must test only free, unbound, bioavailable testosterone.* Use an inexpensive saliva kit ($85 for both testosterone and DHEA).

The youthful ideal for men is about 100 on the ZRT saliva scale, and women should be about 30 on the ZRT scale. Most all men over the age of 50 will have a result of about 50. Women can be too high or too low. You can also use an online lab for $50.

All saliva and blood results differ; there is no universal standard. Women need a ballpark dose of 150 mcg of testosterone in their blood if they are low. This means a sublingual (or DMSO) dose of 200 mg of enanthate or other common salt, (which contains about 150 mcg of actual testosterone). Men need about 4 mg of enanthate or other common salt sublingually (or in DMSO), which contains about 3 mg of actual testosterone. Pharmacists are not allowed to make DMSO solutions, but you can make them yourself.

Men can add 325 drops (10 ml) of 99 percent DMSO to a 10 X 250 bottle of testosterone enanthate. This is a 20 month supply if you use one drop every morning. Women can add 1,250 drops (39 ml) of 99 percent DMSO to a 1 X 250 bottle. This is a 40 month supply. You can legally buy testosterone online for personal use from offshore pharmacies.

Transdermal creams and gels generally only deliver about 20 percent into your blood. This means 80 percent is wasted. Injections are insanity. Oral testosterone is not absorbed. Nasal sprays are not legal, even by prescription. Compounding pharmacists can provide overpriced sublingual drops, or you can make them up yourself. Men can add 10 ml of vegetable oil to a 10 X 250 bottle of testosterone enanthate. Women can add 39 ml to a 1 X 250 bottle. Use one drop every morning.

CONCLUSION

Just remember, all your hormones work together as a team, in concert, harmoniously like a symphony orchestra. You need to test and balance all your basic hormones as much as possible, to maintain youthful levels throughout your life. This is a pillar of natural health.

15. Heart and Artery Health Review

This chapter will review what we've just covered in the context of total heart and artery health, and not just the pumping pressures of our blood. Yes, hypertension is the most common medical condition in the world. There are many other heart and artery illnesses though.

A full 83 percent of people over 65 years of age die of some form of heart and artery illness. Sixty-eight million Americans have some form of heart disease. Heart attacks, the most common condition, are basically caused by atherosclerosis or clogged arteries. Stroke is the second most common CHD illness.

We have about 1.8 million outright heart attacks every year in the U.S., and almost one-third of those people die. *The real point is that most all of this is avoidable and preventable with better diet and lifestyle.*

RISK FACTORS

Only in the last 45 years, since 1965, has the concept of "risk factors" been studied and accepted. In every country on earth, the biggest killer of humans by far is coronary heart disease. This is especially true in countries like Russia and the former Russian republics. High consumption of animal foods, saturated fats, too many calories, excessive sugars, refined foods, alcohol, caffeine, and nicotine are the main factors. Rich countries are always the sickest countries, despite the elaborate medical care. The sickest people are always the most affluent.

Blood Pressure

Blood pressure is one of the most important risk factors. *The most prominent medical condition in the world!* This entire book has shown how to lower blood pressure naturally. People over 65 sometimes have a condition of high systolic-only blood pressure with a systolic reading of 160 or higher, but a near normal diastolic of 90 or less. You must keep your pressures at 120/80 or lower.

Total Cholesterol

Your *Total Cholesterol* (TC) should be about 150. Yes, that is a practical level if you're not eating meat, poultry, eggs, or dairy. Rural Asians routinely have such levels. *TC is the single most important indicator of CHD health.*

American adults, on average, have high levels of about 240. People who tell you, "cholesterol doesn't count" are obviously totally wrong. Look at Table 15.1 from the MRFIT Study, page 105, to prove this beyond any doubt. This involved over a third of a million real men, and cannot be disputed. You want high levels of high density cholesterol (HDL) and low levels of low density (LDL) cholesterol. You really do not need to be overly concerned with your HDL and LDL, as only diet and lifestyle are going to optimize them.

Some self-appointed "experts" tell you that low cholesterol is bad for you. Billions of Asians prove quite the opposite. *The ideal is 150,* and science has proven this repeatedly. Some elderly, sickly people are unable to make much cholesterol, despite their high fat diets. In such cases, low levels are meaningless. *CHD disease rates fall 2 percent for every 1 percent drop in TC.* That is impressive.

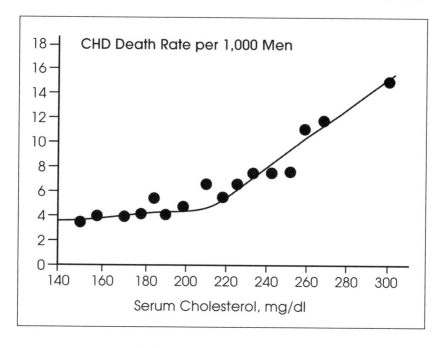

Table 15.1 The MRFIT Study

Triglycerides

Triglycerides are a secondary, but very important indicator of CHD health, and should be under 100 mg/dL (which stands for milligrams per deciliter). All simple sugars and sugar substitutes are the main cause of high triglycerides. Americans commonly have levels of 150, due mostly to their intake of 160 pounds each year of sugars in some form. Fat and sugar work synergistically in our bodies to raise triglyerides. This is why vegetarians often have high triglycerides but low cholesterol; most all of them are sugar addicts.

Homocysteine

Homocysteine is a very accurate and proven marker of CHD health in general. This should be under 10 mmol (is one thousandths of a mole), and preferably well under 10. You must test this.

C-reactive Protein

C-reactive protein (high-sensitivity CRP) is a time-proven inflammation marker for heart and artery health. You must keep this under 3 mg/dl on a 1.0 to 3.0 scale.

Uric Acid

Uric acid is only elevated by eating animal protein from meat, poultry, eggs, and dairy. Your level should be under 5 mg/dl. In addition to cholesterol and triglycerides, be sure to test homocysteine, CRP, and uric acid during your annual physical.

Blood Sugar, Insulin, and Insulin Resistance

Blood sugar, insulin, and *insulin resistance* are very powerful influences on CHD. Fasting insulin should be 5.0 µU/ml or less. Your fasting blood sugar must be *85 or less;* 85 is the Magic Number, not the usual figure of 100 that the doctor will tell you. You should also test your fasting serum insulin. Get an inexpensive GTT test rather than test insulin levels per se. Use a standard 10 points lower than the accepted Western one. You can now buy HbA1c kits in the drugstore for $30. You want a 4.6 percent HbA1c or less, to equal 85 mg/dL blood sugar. This gives you a six month average of glycation (glucose bonding).

Age, Race, And Genetics

Age itself is one of the most important of these factors. The older you are, the more heart and artery disease you'll have. *Race and genetics* are other unchangeable factors. White Europeans are the most prone to heart disease. It is well known that you are more prone if either of your parents had heart disease. Age, genetics, and race are givens.

Anyone over the age of 50, or who suspects any heart problem at all, should seriously consider an inexpensive, noninvasive electrocardiogram (EKG/ECG). This should be standard procedure for this age group. It will reveal hidden and unsuspected problems, especially left ventricular hypertrophy. This is well worth doing and not expensive.

Hormones

Hormones are far more important to heart health than the medical profession realizes. Our endocrine system strongly influences our heart and artery functions. These are discussed in Chapter 13: Your Basic Hormones. The medical profession still holds onto the irrational myth that testosterone is heart unhealthy, while estrogen is heart healthy. Quite the opposite is true, as we've shown. Men do have more heart disease, and women do live six years longer than men on average. It will continually be emphasized that all our hormones work together in harmony, synergistically together as a team. We have fourteen basic hormones that should be balanced, especially after the age of 40. We know youthful levels of T3, T4, testosterone, and DHEA support good CHD health. High levels of estradiol and estrone, on the other hand, are unhealthy. Our other hormones may not have as much direct influence, but *it is just as important to balance them as part of the whole hormone team.* Science will soon prove their value in heart and artery health, too.

Hormones are a happy team, working together in harmony.

DIET AND LIFESTYLE

A healthy diet and lifestyle, together, are crucial in keeping your heart strong and your arteries clear.

Diet

Transfats (aka hydrogenated fats), deserve special mention. Fortunately these have mostly been banned in many countries. You must avoid all hydrogenated fats and oils. These are synthetic chemical creations that clog your arteries. Science has proven that they should never be fed to humans or animals.

The University of Kuopio in Finland fed people a mere 5

percent hydrogenated oil in their food for only a month. They found serious negative effects, especially with cholesterol and triglycerides. Tufts University in Boston, Wegeningen University in the Netherlands, and the University of Oslo are among the hundreds of clinics internationally that have verified this. Harvard Medical School said, *"Hydrogenated fats are directly related to risk of CHD."* Consumption of these has also been clearly connected to various cancer rates.

Margarine is far worse than butter. Read your labels, and never buy or eat anything that contains these chemical abominations. Only eat 10 to 20 percent fat calories, and only from vegetables. *Read your labels.*

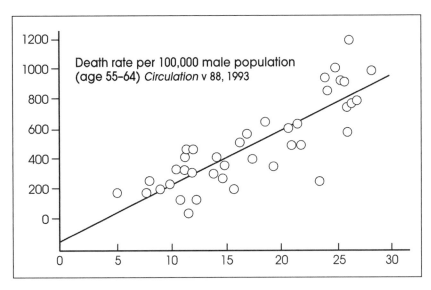

Table 15.2. Cholesterol Saturated Fat Index per 1,000 kcal/day
(The more saturated fat you eat the more coronary heart disease you get based on 40 countries.)

Look at Table 15.2 to prove that the more animal fat you eat the more heart disease you get. This was discussed in Chapter 5: Diet, Diet, Diet. Your worst enemy here, is animal fat and animal protein. *Fat intake must be limited to 10 percent to 20 percent and no more.* This should all be vegetable oils ideally, and not animal fats. Use such oils as sunflower, safflower, corn, and olive, in moderation. Avoid canola oil (there are no canola plants!), as it is another chemical aberration full of toxic erucic acid. If you insist on eating meat, poultry, or eggs you must limit these to 10 percent of your diet or one four-ounce serving a day. Dairy should be omitted completely, even the low-fat and no-fat varieties.

Proven *supplements* are very important, but secondary to diet. The supplements were discussed in Chapter 8: Proven Supplements. If you are over 40, take most all of these for total holistic health. *Treat your whole body and not just your cardio-vascular system.* The most important heart healthy supplements are beta-sitosterol, vitamins, minerals, flax oil, vitamin D, and soy isoflavones.

Obesity

Obesity is very closely related to heart and artery diseases rates. There is abdominal "male" obesity and hips/buttocks "female" obe-sity. Americans eat twice the calories they need, eight times the fat they need (42 percent), the worst kinds of fats, 160 pounds of various sugars we don't need at all, refined foods, chemi-calized, colored, and preserved foods. It's not just that obesity causes higher rates of CHD, but that it causes sky-rocketing medical costs, poor quality of life, and much earlier death. *Obe-sity is a major cause of all-cause mortality.* Overweight people live short lives.

Obesity is correlated with every known medical condition and illness (except osteoporosis). This is agreed on by the inter-national scientists. One typical example is Tohuku University in Japan. Studies found statistically significant relationships between excess body weight and increased medical costs, all cause mortality, and increased risk of cancer incidence. Obesity equals a poor-quality short life.

Fasting

Fasting is the most powerful healing method known to man. Fasting one day a week, from dinner to dinner on a given day, is very effective in that you get fifty-two short fasts every year. You can also join our monthly Young Again two-day fast, on the last weekend of every month. Fasting will strengthen your heart and help clear your arteries. Some excellent books on fasting have been written.

Exercise

Exercise has to be emphasized. We all know exercise is heart healthy, but most people don't get nearly enough of it. Most Westerners do not do physical labor anymore, but rather more sedentary, technical jobs. You can do resistance or aerobic, ideally both of these.

Over 30 years ago Nathan Pritikin put very sickly heart patients on a low fat, near-macrobiotic diet based on whole grains. He had them walk as much as they safely could. He got miracles from this simple two step regimen! If he were alive today, used fasting, and had the hormones and supplements we have now, he would get even faster and more dramatic miracles.

Walking is the best and most practical exercise of all. The ideal is to join a gym and go three times a week. Learn to "super-set" and do 50 sets of weights in twenty minutes. This will raise your beta endorphins as well. Endorphins are our "feel good" hormones.

Other Factors

Diabetes has more bad effects than any other illness. The American Diabetes Association defines this as a blood sugar level of 126 mg/dl or higher. That figure is far too high. Even a level of 100 is extremely dangerous. *One in three American children will grow up diabetic.* This is hard to even comprehend. You want an 85 or less blood sugar level.

Smoking is a very powerful contributor to CHD deaths. Male smokers have ten times the basic heart disease rate and women five times. It is estimated that one-third of the heart attacks every year are largely due to smoking.

Drinking *alcohol* in excess of two drinks a day has a negative effect, but none if less than that. However, even two drinks a day causes other health problems. Coffee, or caffeine in any form, raises blood sugar dramatically and causes insulin resistance. *Do not drink even one cup of coffee or an energy drink a day.*

CONCLUSION

It should be emphasized that lowering any of these factors with prescription drug therapy does not reduce CHD rates at all. Those must be improved with diet and lifestyle. Taking statin drugs does not lengthen life, but it does make your overall health worse. The side effects are very serious. Taking antihypertensive drugs will superficially lower your blood pressure, but it will not add to the years you live. Americans take more prescription drugs than any other country.

16. Bad Habits

One of the *Seven Steps to Natural Health* (listed on page 119) is to limit or stop any bad habits. One doesn't have to be a saint, but you do have to be sincere. You don't have to live the life of an ascetic, but you just can't indulge in whatever you like to do. Freedom is doing the right thing, not doing what you feel like doing.

The bad habits come down to sugar addiction, alcohol, nicotine, caffeine, prescription drugs, and recreational drugs. Yes, taking prescription drugs is a bad habit, too. There is a huge volume of literature on the first four, but there is very little on marijuana, cocaine, ecstasy, amphetamines, or opiates. One of the *Seven Steps to Natural Health* is no prescription drugs; this includes recreational ones as well. Marijuana is anything but innocuous.

BAD HABITS

When you actually realize how harmful sugar, alcohol, nicotine, caffeine, prescription and most recreational drugs are, you will stop using or abusing them. Bad habits just encourage more bad habits. Success breeds success, and failure breeds failure.

Alcohol

The most destructive drug in the entire world is alcohol. People of European descent are the most resistant to alcohol damage, while Asians, Blacks, Latinos, American Indians, and others are far more susceptible to the effects.

The more alcohol you drink, the higher you can expect your blood pressure to go. Alcoholics have inordinately high rates. When they stop drinking, their pressures immediately drop significantly and stay lower. Studies in the *Lancet* (v 1, 1984), *Hypertension* (v 44, 2004 and v 9, 1987) and the book *Hypertension* (Klatsky 2000) all show very clearly that there is a direct correlation between how much alcohol you drink and how high your pressures are.

There is no "French Paradox!" Alcohol is proven to cause liver damage and many other problems. Some studies have shown that eliminating alcohol is more important than exercise. At Kyushi University, it was found that even light drinking raised blood pressure in Japanese people. At Yamagata University, alcohol response was shown to be a largely genetic factor. Epidemiological studies over the last quarter-century prove beyond any doubt the relationship of alcohol intake and hypertension, especially heavier drinking. Blood pressure falls within days of alcohol cessation of alcohol, and it rises within days when it is resumed.

A study in the *American Journal of Clinical Nutrition* (v 87, 2008) found alcohol clearly contributed to metabolic syndrome or pre-diabetes. The more alcohol people consumed the more prone to diabetes and insulin resistance they were. At the University of Barcelona (*Hypertension* v 33, 1999), men who drank over 100 g (about 3.3 oz) of pure ethanol daily were admitted to their clinic, where they stopped drinking. In one month their systolic pressure fell an average of 7.2 mm, and their diastolic fell 6.6 mm. Their heart rate also decreased significantly. On admission, 42 percent were diagnosed with clinical hypertension, but after only 30 days this fell to 12 per cent. This is amazing. It was done with no change in diet or exercise, but just the elimination of all alcohol. The University of Texas verified these findings (*Hypertension* v 39, 2002).

Let's be clear, *alcohol is a biological poison,* and ideally you should never drink at all. Yes, the ideal is no alcohol. Even one drink a day will hurt you, and this is especially true of women. Women are far more sensitive to alcohol damage than men.

Just three or more drinks daily for men and two or more drinks for women are considered "heavy" drinking. Drinking also contributes to obesity, and obesity is another very basic factor here. All these are well established, inarguable facts. Alcohol never improved anyone's life.

Caffeine

It seems the entire world is addicted to the caffeine in coffee and tea. *Caffeine is the most popular psychoactive drug in the world!* It is an insidiously addictive drug. The explosion of energy drinks in the last few years has greatly expanded the use of caffeine, especially among younger people. The documented side effects of caffeine include panic attacks, seizures, tremors, psychosis, vomiting, anxiety, sleep disorders, rapid heart rate, impotence, digestive damage, and a long list of other serious medical conditions.

At Okayama University, the researchers found that caffeine is an angiotensin blocker, and it increases blood pressure 5 to 10 mmHg. At the University of Oklahoma, the doctors warned that caffeine is an important contributor to the extreme incidence of hypertension in our country, and it should be curtailed. Caffeine raises blood pressure by elevating vascular resistance. The pressor response (increase in arterial blood pressure) to caffeine occurs equally in persons at rest and under stress. Again, at this university caffeine was given to five distinct hypertension groups. Caffeine raised both systolic and diastolic blood pressure in all groups."

The largest study of all, from the University of Helsinki, studied 24,710 healthy Finnish people, not on hypertensive drugs or with any known CHD conditions. The results indicated that *coffee drinking increases the risk of hypertensive drug treatment,* and this risk was higher in subjects with low-to-moderate coffee intakes. We get the same results from the Israeli Hypertension Institute, Duke University, and other clinics.

The most comprehensive study came from the University of Utrect. Coffee abstinence was associated with a lower hypertension risk than was low coffee consumption. *Even one cup a day has strong negative effects.* All the above equally applies to the $20 billion a-year energy drinks.

Prescriptive Drugs

Americans take far more prescription drugs than anyone else. The most popular are Vicodin®, prednisone (inflammation), antibiotics, gabapentin (seizures), lisinopril (hypertension), lipitor (cholesterol), metformin (diabetes), anti-depressants, anti-anxiety, and sleep medications.

Yes, Vicodin® (hydrocodeine) is the most prescribed drug in America, with over 100 million prescriptions a year. One in four American women over the age of 50 is on some kind of psych drug. Now school children are routinely given amphetamines (Adderall and Ritalin) to control them.

This total overuse of prescription drugs is epidemic in America. There is just no reason to take prescription drugs, except temporarily in emergencies (and rare cases, such as insulin for type 1 diabetics). The regular use of toxic, synthetic, chemical poisons will only make your health problems worse. You cannot poison your way to health obviously.

Recreational and Non-prescription Drugs

Recreational, non-prescription drug use is also an epidemic. Opiates, especially heroin, fentanyl, and oxycodeine, are an epidemic now.

Marijuana is all too popular among people of all ages, and it will soon be fully legalized. Yes, marijuana has physical side effects. It also causes psychological and mental deterioration, including apathy, lack of motivation, forgetfulness, and mental fogginess.

Ecstasy is a modified amphetamine, and is toxic. Amphetamine and methamphetamine users become dependent, and ruin their bodies, their minds, and their very lives.

Cocaine is as addictive as it is overrated—*the drug of illusion*. In countries like Peru, where it is legal, people drink coca tea. They are as dependent as people are dependent on coffee, but there is no antisocial or criminal activity associated with it since it is legal. Cocaine use has been strongly associated with hypertension and heart disease in general.

Psychedelics largely went out of favor after the early 1970s. There is almost no biological damage here, but the mental effects from them are powerful, mostly all due to insincere use. Dependence on anything harms you.

Sugar Addiction

The main bad habit is sugar addiction. Americans gulp down over 160 pounds of various sugars and sugar substitutes every year. This is an addiction, plain and simple. This insane intake of sugars causes high blood sugar and insulin resistance. *Insulin resistance and blood sugar dysfunction is the key to understanding hypertension*. Sugars and sugar substitutes are the basic cause of blood sugar disorders of all types.

You don't need sweeteners in your diet. Honey is no better than white sugar. Sugar substitutes are worse than natural sugars. Ten per cent fresh (or frozen) fruit is all you can safely eat, and many people should just stop eating fruit altogether. Fruit simply just has no real nutrition to speak of, and fruit is basically sugar, water, and a little fiber. There are almost no minerals or vitamins in any fruit. Read the article *Fruits Have Almost No Nutrition* on our website.

Tobacco

There is very little information about the use of tobacco and nicotine on blood pressure. Some studies found it raised pressure, while other studies actually found a lowering effect.

The doctors at Dongguk University in South Korea claimed cigarette smoking acutely increases arterial stiffness and blood pressure in male smokers with hypertension, and the effects persist longer than in male smokers without hypertension.

The San Diego campus of the University of California showed that smoking clearly raises homocysteine levels (9.5 vs 7.9 mmol). Oestra Hospital in Sweden claimed that smokers had significantly lower systolic (but not diastolic) blood pressures. The Centre de Recherche Clinique said that even former smokers have definitely higher rates of hypertension than never smokers.

CONCLUSION

Freedom is not doing what you want, but doing what is best. Will power is an illusion, and no amount of imagined "will power" is going to stop you from bad habits. *Insight is the key.* Understanding brings freedom from bad habits.

Seven Steps
to Natural Health

With these seven steps you can cure "incurable" illnesses like cancer, diabetes, heart disease, and others naturally without drugs, surgery, or chemotherapy. These are seven vital steps to take if you want optimum health and long life. Do your best to do all of them. The only step to add would be prayer or meditation.

1. An American macrobiotic whole grain based diet is central to everything. Diet cures disease; everything else is secondary.

2. Proven supplements are powerful when you're eating right. There are only about seventeen scientifically proven supplements for those over forty, and eight for those under forty.

3. Natural hormone balance is the third step. Your basic hormones are listed on page 85. You can do this easily and inexpensively without a doctor.

4. Exercise is vital, even if it is just a half-hour of walking a day. Whether it is aerobic or resistance you need to exercise regularly.

5. Fasting is the most powerful healing method known to man. Just fast from dinner to dinner on water one day a week. Join

our monthly Young Again two day fast. The fasting calendar is at www.youngagain.org the last weekend of every month.

6. No prescription drugs, except *temporary* antibiotics or pain medication during an emergency. (There are rare exceptions, such as insulin for type 1 diabetics who have no operant pancreas.)

7. The last step is to end any bad habits, such as alcohol, coffee, nicotine, recreational drugs, or desserts. You don't have to be a saint, but you do need to be sincere.

With these seven steps you can cure "incurable" illnesses naturally like cancer, diabetes, heart disease, and others without drugs, surgery, or radiation. In the entire course of human history, we have never had these seven steps available to us. Affirmative prayer can be your eighth step. Read the article *Affirmative Prayer* at our website.

About the Author

Roger Mason is an internationally known research chemist who studies natural health and longevity. He has written ten different unique and cutting edge books about his findings. He sold Beta Prostate® in 2011, walked away from radio and TV, and formed a charitable trust. He lives with his wife and dog in Wilmington, NC, where they run Young Again Products. You can get his free weekly health newsletter, read his 10 books, and 150 articles for free at www.youngagain.org.

Index

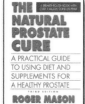

THE NATURAL PROSTATE CURE
THIRD EDITION
Roger Mason

This book provides a unique and effective alternative to risky prostate surgery and drug therapies. The book opens with a basic lesson in proper diet and presents the best supplements for maintaining a healthy prostate, including beta-sitosterol, a vital key to prostate well-being. The author then talks about steps that can be taken to cure prostate disease, including cancer. Finally, the author discusses how hormone imbalances are a major factor contributing to prostate issues. The last chapters of the book suggest hormone treatments that can prevent and combat these conditions.

$9.95 US • 144 pages • 6 x 9-inch quality paperback • ISBN 978-0-7570-0476-6

LOWER YOUR CHOLESTEROL WITHOUT DRUGS, SECOND EDITION
Roger Mason

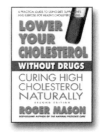

According to the AHA, high cholesterol is the leading cause of coronary heart disease, which continues to be the #1 killer in North America. While millions of Americans take prescription medications to lower their cholesterol, the fact is, these drugs often have very dangerous side effects. In his updated edition of *Lower Your Cholesterol Without Drugs,* author Roger Mason offers you safe and natural alternatives to effectively lower your cholesterol levels. He does so in a no-holds-barred manner, separating the fairy tales from the scientifically valid truths.

$9.95 US • 128 pages • 6 x 9-inch quality paperback • ISBN 978-0-7570-0481-7

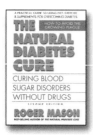

THE NATURAL DIABETES CURE
SECOND EDITION
Roger Mason

Poor nutrition is the major cause of blood sugar disorders like diabetes, but most people don't know how to maintain a healthy, balanced diet. In *The Natural Diabetes Cure,* Roger Mason provides an effective nutritional approach to preventing and combating diabetes. The book begins by explaining how the condition develops, and then details how a diet of whole grains and vegetables can greatly improve overall health. Additional chapters discuss nutritional supplements that can help regulate blood sugar, and explore important topics such as hormone balance and exercise.

$9.95 US • 128 pages • 6 x 9-inch quality paperback • ISBN 978-0-7570-0369-1

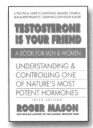

TESTOSTERONE IS YOUR FRIEND

THIRD EDITION

Roger Mason

Testosterone is responsible for stimulating and controlling "masculine" characteristics like muscles and hair growth. What many people don't realize is that this hormone is present to a lesser degree in females. What's more, low testosterone levels can cause countless health problems for both sexes, including memory loss, anxiety and depression, osteoporosis, increased cholesterol levels, weight gain, sexual dysfunction, and infertility. While testosterone supplements are available, most are ineffective and some are dangerous. In this book, Roger Mason presents the latest and most effective natural treatments and supplements to help raise testosterone levels.

$9.95 US • 128 pages • 6 x 9-inch quality paperback • ISBN 978-0-7570-0477-3

NATURAL HEALTH FOR WOMEN

SECOND EDITION

Roger Mason

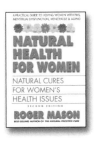

When hormones are not produced in the proper amounts or they are not in balance, a number of health problems can occur. Symptoms of hormonal imbalance can range from mild cramping, irritability, and food cravings to hot flashes and night sweats—along with more serious conditions, such as osteoporosis, diabetes, and cancer. Standard HRTs are often used to correct hormonal problems; but they can have dangerous side effects. In this newly revised book, Roger Mason offers naturally effective alternatives to help keep hormones in balance.

$9.95 US • 160 pages • 6 x 9-inch quality paperback • ISBN 978-0-7570-0368-4

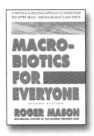

MACROBIOTICS FOR EVERYONE, SECOND EDITION

Roger Mason

Making the right food choices is not always a priority. We may be considered an educated society, yet seem to be blind to the fact that our diets are typically unhealthy—low in whole grains, legumes, and fresh produce, and high in processed, fat-laden, sugary foods and beverages. This unwholesome diet puts us at risk for such serious health conditions as heart disease, arthritis, diabetes, and cancer. In *Zen Macrobiotics for Everyone*, Roger Mason makes healthy eating fun, delicious, and, most important, easy.

$9.95 US • 128 pages • 6 x 9-inch quality paperback • ISBN 978-0-7570-0372-1

**For more information about our books,
visit our website at www.squareonepublishers.com**